The House Mouse

Karl Theiler

The House Mouse

Atlas of Embryonic Development

With a Foreword by Heiner Westphal

With 335 Illustrations

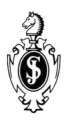

Springer Science+Business Media, LLC

Dr. Karl Theiler
Department of Anatomy, University of Zurich, Winterthurerstrasse 190,
CH-8057 Zurich, Switzerland

Library of Congress Cataloging-in-Publication Data
Theiler, Karl.
    The house mouse : atlas of embryonic development / Karl Theiler.
        p.   cm.
    Bibliography: p.
    Includes index.
    ISBN 978-3-642-88420-7
    1. Mice — Development — Atlases.   2. Embryology — Mammals — Atlases.
I. Title.
QL937.T45   1989
599.32′33 — dc19   88-24888

Typeset by Publishers Service, Bozeman, Montana.
9 8 7 6 5 4 3 2
ISBN 978-3-642-88420-7   ISBN 978-3-642-88418-4 (eBook)
DOI 10.1007/978-3-642-88418-4

Foreword

During the Middle Ages, precious books used to be chained to the walls of libraries so that nobody would carry them off. I wish we could do that with our cherished first edition of Theiler's book (the only one I could find at the NIH), which we fondly call our mouse bible.

The molecular biology of the mouse has taken center stage because of the advent of transgenic technology, which allows us to observe specific genes at work in the developing mammalian organism. Molecular biologists are in dire need for education in each and every aspect of the biology of the mouse, not the least of which is its anatomy.

With unparalleled accuracy resulting from a lifelong devotion to anatomical detail, Karl Theiler has created a description of the developmental stages of the mouse that has become widely accepted as a standard reference compendium. Springer-Verlag is to be highly commended for making this book available once again for a new generation of researchers eager to learn about the genes that regulate this beautiful unfolding of a complex living organism from a one-cell embryo.

HEINER WESTPHAL, MD
Head, Section on Mammalian Gene Regulation
Laboratory of Molecular Genetics
National Institute of Child Health
and Human Development
National Institutes of Health
Bethesda, Maryland

Preface

Detailed photographs of different stages of mouse embryos have become increasingly important for current research involving the use of transgenic mice. The description of the development of the laboratory mouse, "The House Mouse," being out of print, a re-edition seemed to be desirable. The original series of photographs was still available. The text needed only some minor changes. In the bibliography, a restricted selection of recent papers has been added; completeness was not intended in view of the availability of computerized lists of publications in some libraries.

KARL THEILER

Contents

Introduction

The external form typical of each age group is represented by profile photographs, and there is a short description of characteristic features. Some organs, such as the eye, ear, and pituitary and pineal gland, are particularly useful for determining stages in development. These are described in more detail. To complete the picture of the structural organization as a whole, graphic reconstructions were made.

Any subdivision of development into stages must necessarily be arbitrary. I have tried to use as a guide the classification of Streeter [6] in his "Developmental horizons of human embryos," and I have pointed out equivalent human-mouse stages [4] whenever possible. For older human embryos, I have used the age data of Olivier and Pineau [*Bull. Ass. Anat.* 47, 573–576 (1962)]. This classification is restricted to initial organogenesis, and precise comparisons in staging between human and mouse cannot be made. Some phases of development are faster in the mouse than in the human, and some are slower. For practical reasons, in this text, both stage number and age in days will be given together. The chapter numbers also correspond to the stage numbers.

The reference list is subdivided under various headings. It is brief and emphasizes recent investigations. No references on the rat are included, and the author apologizes for the inevitable incompleteness.

Materials and Methods

To obtain hybrid embryos, females of our inbred C57BL/6 stock were crossed, at the age of 3–5 months, with CBA males. Usually first litters were used, but a few second litters were included.

Strains. C57BL/6 Th, F? + 20, transferred to Zurich in 1960 from The Jackson Laboratory, Bar Harbor, Maine. CBA F? + 10, also received in 1960 from The Jackson Laboratory. The nomenclature of inbred strains is explained in *J. Heredity* 54, 159–162, 1963, and in Green [2].

Procedure

Animals were placed in a room in which the normal light-dark sequence was reversed for at least 4 days. Three or four females were placed with a male in total darkness. Copulation was determined by the presence of a vaginal plug. The middle of the "artificial night" was designated as day 0 of pregnancy. It is not considered identical with ovulation time. A late ovulation may result in considerable retardation in development. On the other hand, an early ovulation does not advance development, because the second maturation division is completed only after fertilization.

For each period several litters were examined. The most advanced embryos were regarded as representative of the respective age groups. If by chance all litters of one group stem from especially early or late ovulations, a difference from the "developmental curve" would result. When this was observed, additional litters were obtained for this group. For the first 3 days, successive stages were designated a full day apart. Days 4 to 12 were designated a half day apart. The 12-hour staging regularly revealed an overlapping of developmental phases.

Some specimens were fixed in Bouin's solution, 4% formol, or Carnoy's solution, and imbedded in paraffin. Some early embryos were fixed in OsO_4 and embedded in Methacrylate to prepare thin sections.

The serial sections were routinely stained with Hematoxylin-Eosin (H.-E.). Additional information was gained by the use of periodic-acid-Schiff-reaction. Older specimens were stained with azocarmine-aniline blue. Cleared skeletons were stained with alizarin-red S or methylgreen.

Stage 1   One-celled Egg
1–20 Hours

Human equivalent
Horizon I, one-celled egg

Stage 1 begins with *fertilization*. It invariably occurs in the ampulla tubae, the dilated uppermost loop of the coiled oviduct (Fig. 1). *The eggs*, after ovulation, are in the metaphase stage of the second maturation division (Fig. 2). They are surrounded by follicle cells, which tend to clump together (Fig. 4). In each ampulla, there are 3 to 5 ova.

After 6 hours the eggs are still encircled by several layers of follicle cells. Sometimes these show mitotic cell divisions, side by side with pycnotic nuclei. Some ova are already fertilized. As an example, the specimen KT 980 contained 9 ova, of which 2 could definitely be regarded as fertilized. No first polar body was seen in any of these cells.

Evidently the first polar body soon becomes cytolized. After ovulation, it is usually no longer visible. However, it may persist in exceptional cases, for instance, as in specimen KT 791, a 2-celled egg of 24 hours.

After 10 hours the eggs are still located in the ampulla tubae. There are fewer follicle cells surrounding them, and many are pycnotic. The percentage of fertilized ova has considerably increased: for example, all of 8 egg cells in specimen KT 982 were fertilized, and all have emitted the second polar body (Fig. 5). All except one contained a male pronucleus (Fig. 6). Chang [11] observed that not even 50% of the eggs in this stage were fertilized.

After 20 hours all follicle cells have disappeared. The eggs are now located between the first and second loop of the oviduct (KT 972). The male pronucleus approaches the female pronucleus and starts mitosis (Figs. 7 and 8). The *zona pellucida* shrinks considerably after fixation in Bouin's solution, so that the overall diameter, in the fixed state, amounts to only 55 to 60 microns.

Overripe eggs are from time to time encountered in the oviduct (KT 995, KT 966). Within the first 10 hours after copulation, they can be easily recognized by the lack of surrounding follicle cells. In one case, a "nude" single egg contained 4 pronuclei of different sizes. Sometimes overripe eggs seem to initiate division, and they consist of several loosely adhering cells with only faintly staining nuclei. Similar degenerating blastomeres often occur in the ovary, within atretic follicles. They may arise by "spontaneous parthenogenesis." Artificial parthenogenesis has been described recently [15].

Material	Age	Content
KT 993/94	2 h	3 eggs in meiosis
KT 966	5 h	Degenerating eggs
KT 995	5 h	6 eggs, some degenerating
KT 979	6 h	Degenerating eggs
KT 980	6 h	9 eggs with female pronucleus, some fertilized
KT 981	10 h	8 eggs in second meiotic division
KT 971/72	20 h	8 eggs: one 2-celled, 1 triploid, 1 degenerating
KT 977/78	20 h	7 eggs: 6 definitely fertilized, with pronuclei and polocytes

Figs. 1–8: Beginning of development, first day

FIG. 1. Overall picture: ovary–oviduct–uterine horn.
A = ampulla tubae, Cl = freshly ruptured follicle, I = infundibulum, O = ostium uterinum tubae, projecting in uterine lumen.
KT 972. 22.5:1

FIG. 2. Tubal egg in second meiotic division, not fertilized, in ampulla.
KT 981. 720:1

FIG. 3. Spermatozoa, epididymal smear, iron-hematoxylin.
R = cytoplasmic droplet at end of mid piece. 1300:1

FIG. 4. Ampulla tubae with 2 fertilized eggs and surrounding follicle cells. 135:1

FIG. 5. Detail, showing sperm head under zona pellucida.
Opposite to it, P indicates polar body, in telophase.
KT 982, 10 h. 720:1

FIG. 6. Male and female pronucleus.
KT 982, 10 h. 720:1

FIG. 7. Male pronucleus approaches and starts mitosis.
Polar body P is detached.
KT 972, 20 h. 900:1

FIG. 8. Both nuclear membranes dissolved. Amphimixis.
KT 978, 20 h. 900:1

4

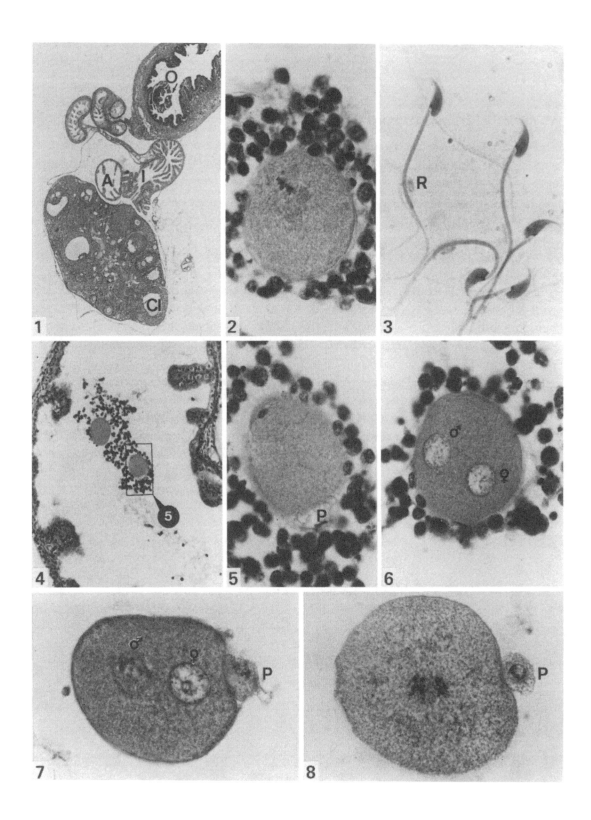

Stage 2   Beginning of Segmentation
20–24 Hours

Within 24 hours the first cleavage division is completed. The eggs are near the exit of the ampulla, between the first and the second loop of the oviduct (Fig. 9). This second loop is said to exhibit peristaltic contractions, which aid ova transport [5]. *The first cleavage* yields two cells of about equal size, with finely granulated cytoplasm. Their large spherical nuclei contain 4–5 nucleoli that are surrounded by a small border of chromatin. The egg and zona pellucida shrink considerably after Bouin's fixation. The overall diameter is 48 to 64 microns, including the zona. After fixation with OsO_4 there is much less shrinkage and the zona appears in sections as a distinct thick ring (Figs. 10 and 11), with an overall diameter of 83 microns. In the fresh, unfixed state, eggs of this stage are 80–100 microns in diameter.

The second polar body is tangentially cut in Fig. 12. The first polar body, visible in another plane of section, is located about 90 degrees from the second, and is in metaphase. The nucleus of the second polocyte is typically small and has peripheral chromatin (Fig. 10).

The corpus luteum has slightly enlarged cells, which form irregular trabeculae separated by invading capillaries. As an exception, in Fig. 9 a distinct central blood coagulum is visible. *Spermatozoa* are visible in the oviduct and uterus up to 20 hours after copulation (KT 975). There are also few leukocytes and other free cells. Thereafter, spermatozoa disappear completely.

Material	Age	Content
KT 975/76	20 h	4 fertilized eggs: one 2-celled, in the process of cleavage, one degenerating
KT 790/91	24 h	4 fertilized eggs: all 2-celled, at lower end of first loop of oviduct
KT 729	45 h	Eggs not fertilized, some exhibiting second meiotic division, some degenerating

Figs. 9–12: Beginning of segmentation, 20 h

FIG. 9. Overall picture: ovary–oviduct.
Drawing (*right*) shows location of eggs in oviduct (*arrow*); *Cl* = fresh corpus luteum. Bouin, H.-E.
KT 791. 40:1

FIG. 10. Two-celled egg with polar body indicated by *P*. Phase contrast. Fixation OsO_4.
KT 790. 270:1

FIG. 11. Two-celled egg.
In nucleus, *N*, several small nucleoli are visible. Phase contrast. Fixation OsO_4.
KT 790. 270:1

FIG. 12. Two-celled egg, higher magnification. Bouin, H.-E.
The zona pellucida obviously thinned in comparison to Figs. 10 and 11.
KT 791. 580:1

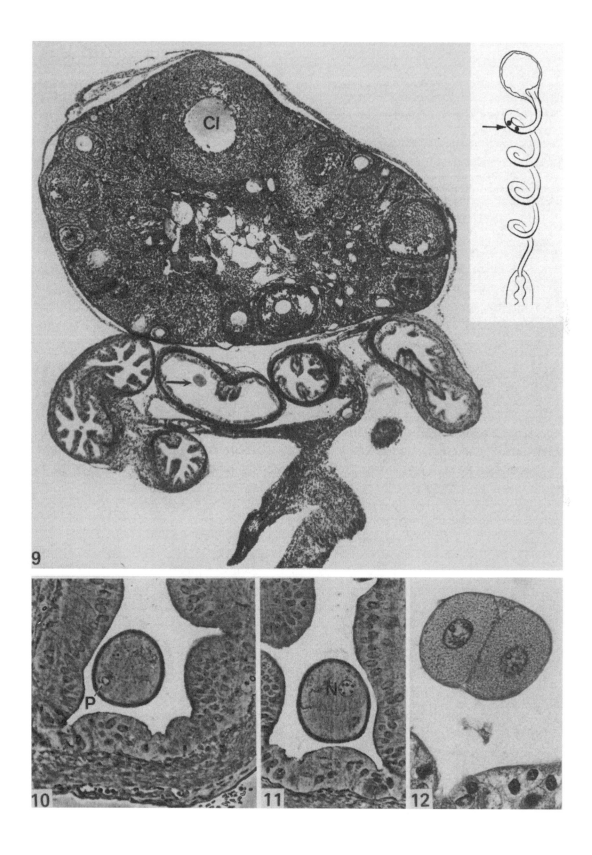

Stage 3 Segmenting Egg
2 Days, Morula

After 52–53 hours the embryos are composed of *2 to 16 cells*. This difference in degree of development must have existed in the previous stage, and is probably a result of different fertilization times.

The *blastomeres* are of unequal size, and some are dividing mitotically. The cytoplasm is finely granulated throughout and the nuclei are rather small. On the other hand, nucleoli enlarge considerably, and their number decreases. In the two-celled egg, 4 or 5 small nucleoli are visible in each cell. In the 4-celled stage, there are only 2 or 3.

A *segmentation cavity* is not yet visible. At the 8-celled stage, the contours of the blastomeres of fresh specimens are no more distinctly visible (stage of compaction): the cells attach close together.

The diameter of the morulae after Bouin fixation is 70 microns (KT 845), including the shrunken *zona pellucida*. The eggs are still in clusters. They have advanced to the lower half of the oviduct.

The polocytes are still present, even in the 16-celled morulae. Their nuclei appear pycnotic.

Corpora lutea measure 700–750 microns. The central cavity is filled by connective tissue and contains little blood and fibrin. Rarely leukocytes are encountered (Fig. 15).

Spermatozoa are no longer visible in the uterus or the oviduct.

Material	Age	Eggs
KT 846	52 h	1 one-celled and 3 four-celled eggs
KT 845	53 h	4 six-celled, 1 nine-celled, and 1 sixteen-celled egg

Figs. 13–17: Cleavage, 53 h

FIG. 13. Corpus luteum, overall picture. Bouin, H.-E.
Drawing (*right*) shows location of eggs in oviduct.
KT 845. 125:1

FIG. 14. Detail of Fig. 13, showing the connective tissue organization of the central region. 360:1

FIG. 15. Detail of the adjacent section.
Arrow indicates leukocytes appearing in connection with the central reorganization. 720:1

FIG. 16. Segmenting egg of 9 cells, with polar body, *P*, in oviduct. Bouin, H.-E.
KT 845. 270:1

FIG. 17. Segmenting egg of 9 cells, median section.
Zona pellucida extremely thin (fixation effect).
KT 845. 760:1

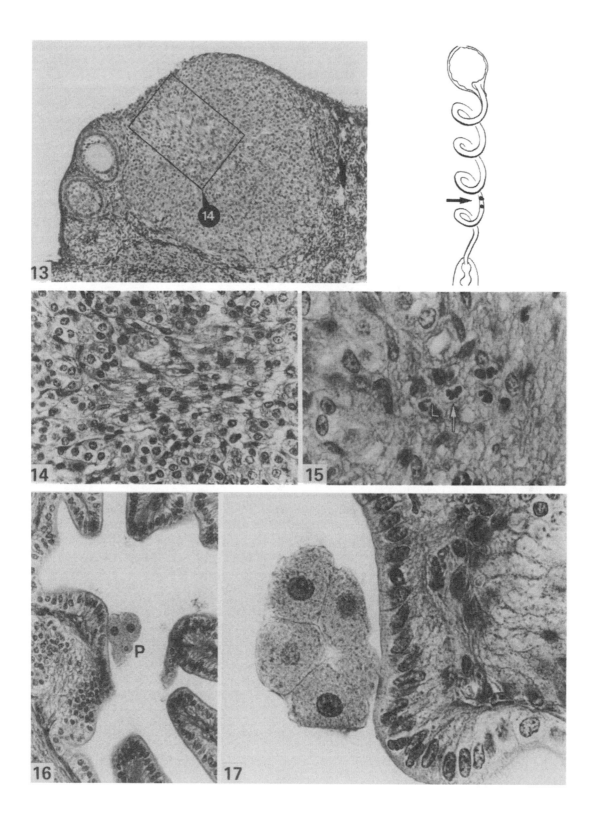

Stage 4   Advanced Segmentation
3 Days

On the third day, the eggs are in the uterus [17]. After 71 hours, one was found in the pars intramuralis tubae (KT 786). The eggs were composed of 16–25 cells after 69–71 hours.

The *blastomeres* are not quite equal in size. The cytoplasm is coarsely granulated, with spherical or rod-like eosinophilic inclusions. The nucleoli are extraordinarily large and may be one-third of the nuclear diameter. Out of 15 nuclei of specimen KT 934:

> 10 showed a single big nucleolus,
> 3 showed two nucleoli of unequal size,
> 2 showed several small nucleoli.

The trophoblast cannot yet be distinguished with certainty from the embryoblast. The segmentation cavity forms very rapidly (78 hours), and makes it possible to distinguish the embryoblast from the trophoblast. The 25-celled egg lacks a distinct cavity, but the 35-celled egg (78 hours) has a large eccentrically placed lumen.

The *diameter* of the morulae has apparently not changed. After fixation in Bouin's solution or Carnoy's solution (which is suitable for a PAS-reaction), it was 62–70 microns. The *zona pellucida* stains intensively red with the PAS reaction.

Polocytes are sometimes still distinct. Their nuclei are pycnotic and slightly larger than the nucleolus of a blastomere. The cytoplasm is PAS-negative.

The *distances* between the eggs have increased, and the eggs are irregularly spaced.

The *corpora lutea* are more intensely vascularized than in the previous stage.

Material	Age	Morulae
KT 786	71 h	18-celled, in pars intramuralis tubae
KT 777	69 h	22-celled, 5 of which are in mitosis, in uterus
KT 934	69 h	1 showing 16 cells, with distinct polocyte
		1 showing 18 cells
		1 showing 20 cells, 2 of which are in mitosis
		1 showing 25 cells, 7 of which are in mitosis
KT 989/90	78 h	2 morulae with 33 and 34 cells, in uterus
		1 blastocyst, 37 cells
KT 991/92	78 h	1 morula, 31 cells
		4 blastocysts: 35, 36, 42, and 43 cells

Figs. 18–22: Cleavage, 69 h

Fig. 18. Low magnification. Uterine horn, cross sectioned. Bouin, H.-E. KT 934. 54:1

Fig. 19. Detail of Fig. 18, with 16-celled morula. Drawing (*right*) shows location of eggs (*arrow*). 360:1

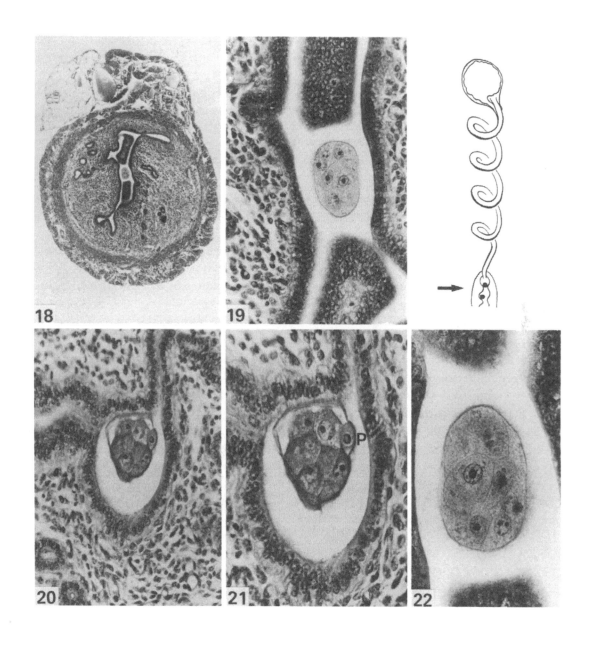

FIG. 20. Morula of 21 cells, Carnoy, PAS.
Distinct zona pellucida, partly separated from blastomeres because of shrinkage. Beginning formation of a crypt in uterine lumen. No deciduous reaction yet.
KT 934. 360:1

FIG. 21. Morula of 21 cells.
Polar body, P, with pycnotic nucleus (not to be confused with a nucleolus).
KT 934a. 560:1

FIG. 22. Morula of 16 cells. Bouin, H.-E.
Nuclei containing one big or two small nucleoli. Zona pellucida very thin (fixation effect).
KT 934. 720:1

11

Horizon III
Free blastocyst

Stage 5   Blastocyst
4 Days

After 100 hours, almost all blastocysts have arrived in the uterus. The only exception was specimen KT 969, where the right oviduct contained 4 probably decaying blastocysts. None had reached the right horn of the uterus. The other uterine horn had 3 normal blastocysts, and the adjoining tube was empty.

The eggs are distinctly spaced along the entire uterus, apparently free within the lumen, sometimes in a crypt. In most cases, the wall of the blastocyst was probably already in close contact with the uterine epithelium, and is secondarily separated by fixation shrinkage (Fig. 29). The *blastocyst* is clearly separated into embryoblast and trophoblast. The trophoblastic cells are flattened, and form a single-layered epithelium. They are said to absorb amino acids, perhaps influenced by hormones [19].

The embryoblastic cells are cuboidal and clustered at the embryonic pole. The nuclei of both trophoblast and embryoblast usually contain an elongated nucleolus [10] with a peripheral border of chromatin; sometimes, additional nucleoli are visible. Each cell invariably shows several chromocenters.

The total number of cell varies. Specimen KT 970/72 consisted of 27 embryonic and 98 trophoblastic cells. In addition, there is an indistinct polocyte adhered to the trophoblast.

Figs. 23–29: Blastocyst, 101 h

FIG. 23. Ovary with 3 corpora lutea, low magnification. PAS.
KT 967. 40:1

FIG. 24. Detail of Fig. 23.
Corpus luteum with enlarged blood vessels. 115:1

FIG. 25. Uterine horn, longitudinal section. Blastocyst (*arrow*) antimesometrial.
M = mesometerial region of uterus with enlarged blood vessels, PAS.
KT 967. 40:1

FIG. 26. Blastocyst and vicinity, H.-E. C = compact layer of endometrium beneath epithelium. Transverse ridges of the epithelium cause a wavy appearance of the surface.
KT 970. 135:1

FIG. 27. Blastocyst of Fig. 26, enlarged.
Em = embryoblast with mitosis. 720:1

FIG. 28. Blastocyst and vicinity, PAS. A crypt has formed.
KT 967. 135:1

FIG. 29. Detail of next section (Fig. 28).
Fine glycogen granules in trophoblast, T, and the adjoining epithelium, U. In between, a free space, evidently formed artifically by shrinkage (the blastocyst must originally have occupied the whole crypt). 560:1

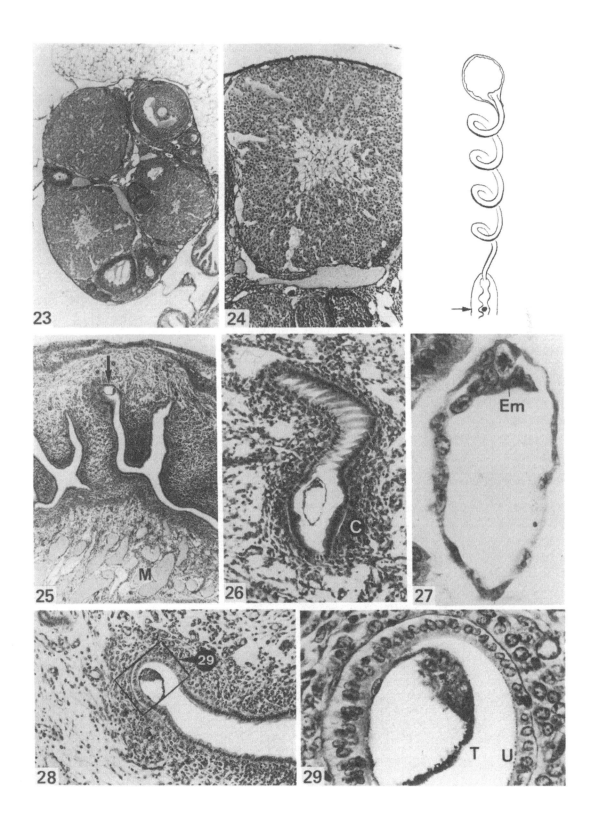

The *zona pellucida* has completely disappeared. The *overall diameter* varies considerably because of deformation, shrinkage and other reasons [13]. For instance, after Carnoy's solution, 2 blastocysts measured 70×100 microns, a third 75×80 microns. The PAS-reaction shows intense red granules within the trophoblastic cells after the zona pellucida disappears (Fig. 29). Some embryoblastic cells bordering the segmentation cavity may contain similar granules, perhaps they represent the first entodermal cells.

Corpora lutea contain radially arranged strands of large clear cells, distinctly different from the smaller interstitial and follicle cells (Figs. 23–24). Blood vessels are abundant and sometimes dilated. Within the interstitium, some small clusters of PAS-positive cells with fine red granules may be observed (Fig. 37). They should not be confused with the intensely red debris of degenerating oocytes.

Material	Age	Blastocysts
KT 964	99 h	2 blastocysts in uterus, without zona pellucida
KT 969/70	101 h	3 blastocysts in left uterine horn
		4 blastocysts in right oviduct
KT 967/68	101 h	4 blastocysts in uterus
KT 923	94 h	None visible, one empty zona pellucida

Stage 6   Implantation
4 1/2 Days

At 120 hours, there are distinct differences in degree of development of embryos within the same litter. Some embryos are *beginning implantation*, i.e., the blastocyst closely adheres to the undamaged uterine epithelium (Fig. 32). In other cases, there is advanced erosion of the mucous membrane. Some 4-day embryos are also closely adhered to the undamaged uterine epithelium, and so the beginning of implantation is estimated to occur at 4 1/2 days.

Embryoblast and trophoblast can easily be discriminated at this stage. Trophoblastic cells are flat, with prominent nuclei. Embryoblastic cells are spherical and have larger nucleoli than the trophoblastic cells. Both types of cells are rich in RNA. They stain intensively with Pyronin, in contrast to the underlying endometrium. The *entoderm cells* are already recognizable as a distinct layer and their cytoplasm appears even darker than other embryonic or trophoblastic cells. The number of cells varies. For example, specimen KT 859 (Fig. 31) consisted of 76 entodermal, 34 formative (embryoblastic) and 133 trophoblastic cells.

Invasion

Erosion of the uterine epithelium usually begins somewhat below the equatorial zone of the blastocyst. The adjoining trophoblastic cells are transformed into *"trophoblastic giant cells"* [2] (Fig. 35). The nuclei become large and spherical. The nucleoli also enlarge, and the cytoplasm forms long slender processes.

These cells are easily distinguished from the large *deciduous cells* that now appear in the vicinity of the implantation cavity [40]. They contain little RNA and much glycogen. In H.-E.-sections, the glycogen is dissolved and characteristic vacuoles are visible (Fig. 35). Adjacent to the zone of glycogen cells (Fig. 34, *D*) mentioned above, there is another girdle of cells consisting mainly of enlarged deciduous cells without glycogen droplets. Some of these cells have exceedingly large nuclei (Fig. 34, *D*). At the periphery, toward the muscle layer, the RNA-content of the endometrium decreases considerably.

Material	Age	Blastocysts
KT 859	117 h	1 free, 3 attached, all in one uterine horn. Entoderm distinct (H.-E.-stained)
KT 873	120 h	3 attached in uterus. Entoderm distinct (methylgreen-pyronin stained)
KT 857	124 h	1 free in uterine horn. Entoderm distinct (H.-E.)

Figs. 30–37: Implantation

FIG. 30. Low magnification of uterus, longitudinal section.
M = mesometrium (oblique section), H.-E.
KT 859. 117 h. 40:1

FIG. 31. Blastocyst, enlarged.
KT 859. 560:1

FIG. 32. Blastocyst, 120 h, Carnoy fixation, phase-contrast.
Little shrinkage.
KT 873. 225:1

FIG. 33. Endometrial reaction. Blastocyst attached, 117 h.
KT 859. 135:1

FIG. 34. Detail from Fig. 33.
G = girdle of glycogen cells, D = zone of large deciduous cells. 360:1

FIG. 35. Invasion, high magnification.
The trophoblastic cell, T, is enlarged, and has penetrated the epithelium. In the connective tissue, glycogen containing cells with typical vacuoles, V, are visible, 117 h. 720:1

FIG. 36. Ovary with 4 corpora lutea, PAS, 117 h.
KT 911. 27:1

FIG. 37. Detail of ovary.
Left: margin of corpus luteum, bordering the interstitial gland with enlarged blood vessels and some intensely PAS-positive cells, P. 270:1

16

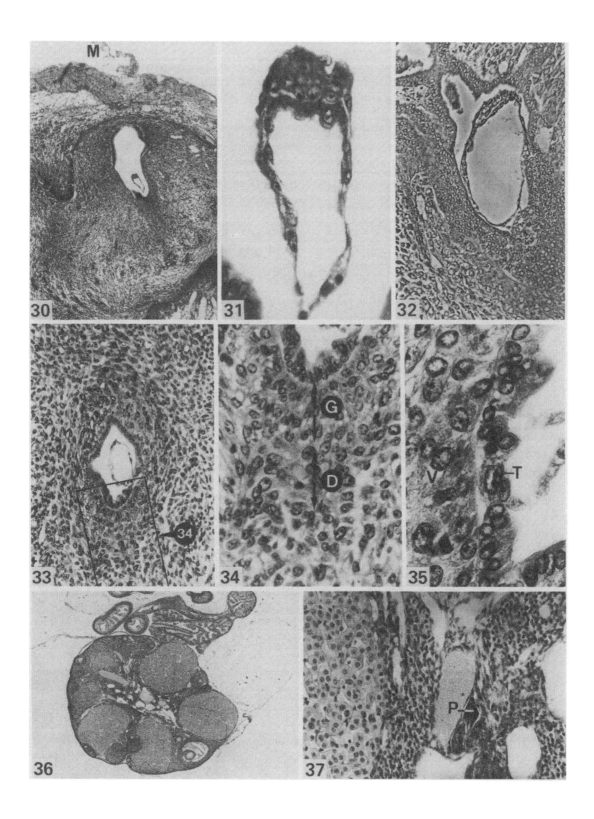

Stage 7   Formation of Egg Cylinder
5 Days

As soon as invasion starts, the embryoblast enlarges considerably and bulges cone-like into the segmentation cavity (Fig. 41). The trophoblast also starts to form an excrescence (trophoblastic cap or ectoplacental cone), which projects above the embryonic pole and stains intensively with H.-E. (Fig. 45).

Embryoblast

The formative cells ("inner cell mass") of the embryoblast may be distinguished from the adjacent "trophoblastic cap" by their pale appearance. The detection of the entodermal cells, on the opposite side of the egg cylinder, is easier. They are cuboidal in shape and have been called proximal or visceral entoderm. Their surface does not appear to be sharply bounded

---

Figs. 38–45: Formation of egg cylinder

FIG. 38. Low magnification of uterus, cross section, PAS, 117 h.
M = mesometrium.
KT 911. 40:1

FIG. 39. Detail: Deciduous reaction.
In the vicinity of the egg, the uterine epithelium is dissolved. Appearance of glycogen cells (dark border) and of large deciduous cells. Enlarged blood vessels, PAS, 117 h. 100:1

FIG. 40. Implantation site enlarged. The uterine epithelium has disappeared.
G = large dark glycogen droplets in glycogen cells, T = trophoblastic giant cell with faintly staining nucleus and large nucleolus, PAS, 117 h. 560:1

FIG. 41. Low magnification of implantation site.
Thin section, OsO_4 fixation, phase-contrast.
KT 782. 360:1

FIG. 42. Detail of Fig. 41.
En = entoblast, with indistinct boundary (because of the presence of microvilli). 900:1

FIG. 43. Detail of Fig. 41.
E = large nucleus of embryonic cell, adjoining uterine epithelium. The latter contains lipoid droplets, sometimes confluent and forming spheres of variable size (L) stained black by OsO_4. 900:1

FIG. 44. Invasion and formation of egg cylinder, H.-E.
KT 693. 120 h. 100:1

FIG. 45. Detail of Fig. 44.
Cap-like thickening of trophoblast, K.
Arrows indicate limits of the uterine epithelium. 270:1

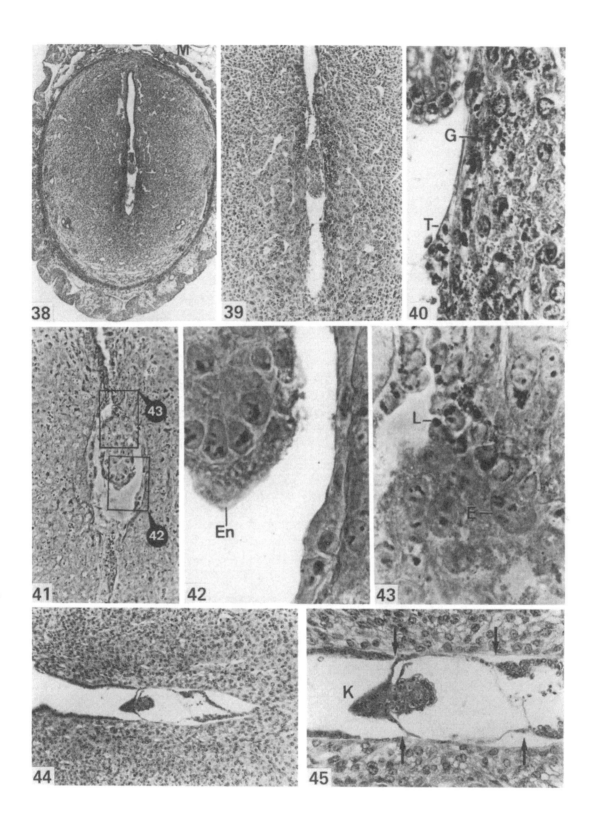

19

with the light microscope because of the presence of microvilli (Fig. 42). Toward the base of the egg cylinder, near the trophoblast, the distinction between embryoblast and trophoblast is less obvious. Some cells migrate along the inner surface of the trophoblast at the base of the egg cylinder (Fig. 45) and become the distal or parietal entoderm.

Trophoblast

Above the egg cylinder the trophoblastic cells are cuboidal in shape and protrude as a cap-like mass (Fig. 45). Further growth of this trophoblastic cap gives rise to the "ectoplacental cone."

The peripheral, flattened trophoblastic cells dissolve the adjacent uterine epithelium. The disintegration proceeds all around the egg cylinder. Within the epithelial cells, large lipoid droplets are often visible (Fig. 43). They have been interpreted as "secretion droplets" [2].

Endometrial Reaction

The endometrial reaction involves both the uterine epithelium and connective tissue [22]. The adjoining epithelial cells degenerate and numerous lipoid droplets form within the cytoplasm. These are stained black with OsO_4 and red with Sudan B.

Fig. 44 shows some cell debris in the original uterine lumen (*right*). In the vicinity of the implantation site, the deciduous cells exhibit a marked glycogen reaction when stained with PAS ("deciduous glycogen cells").

Tubular uterine glands are now more numerous. They are situated in between implantation sites.

Material	Age	
KT 693	119 h	7 egg cylinders, stained with H.-E. Only part of uterus fixed in OsO_4 for thin sections, in methacrylate
KT 782	117 h	2 egg cylinders
KT 911/12	117 h	6 egg cylinders, H.-E. and PAS

Stage 8   Differentiation of Egg Cylinder
6 Days

Implantation sites are easily visible externally as spherical swellings, measuring 2×3 mm (Fig. 46). The spacing of the embryos is now rather regular [26]. However, in one instance, two embryos in one swelling were observed (specimen KT 914).

Embryoblast

The egg cylinder elongates and will soon be divided into *embryonic* and *extraembryonic* areas. In between the two areas there is a small indentation. Soon a central lumen, the *proamniotic cavity* appears, at first in the embryonic region, and later in the extraembryonic area. Most embryos of this stage have already formed a continuous cleft.

Most of the cells of the embryonic ectoderm are cylindrical in shape. They are often separated by a small furrow from the extraembryonic, irregular cuboidal cells.

The entodermal cells become flattened at the ventral end of the egg cylinder. Toward its base, they become cylindrical and accumulate much glycogen in their apical cytoplasm [29] (Fig. 51, *lower left*).

Trophoblast

Trophoblastic cells migrate irregularly from the *ectoplacental cone*, and maternal erythrocytes spill into the developing intercellular lacunae. Ectoplacental cells store much PAS-positive material, probably glycogen (Fig. 51). They are called by Arvis [23] "cellules ultratrophoblastiques." Their shape is more regular than the glycogen cells of the decidua.

The peripheral, previously flattened trophoblastic cells invade the maternal tissue and enlarge greatly. They are often called *primary giant cells* and contain a single, very large nucleus (Fig. 54). The peripheral cells of the ectoplacental cone also begin to enlarge.

Trophoblastic giant cells never undergo mitosis [30]. Their distinction from smaller, so-called "secondary giant cells" [2] (Fig. 107) is perhaps unwarranted as they are also derived from the trophoblast.

Reichert's Membrane

With the appearance of distal (parietal) entoderm, a noncellular thin membrane, Reichert's membrane, forms between the distal entoderm and the peripheral trophoblast (trophectoderm). Though acellular in nature, it increases in size with the growth of the embryo, and can be distinctly recognized during later development. It is secreted by the distal entoderm (see discussion in Green [2]).

Material	Age	Embryos		Lumen (proamnion)	Closure of mesometrial uterine lumen
KT 913/14	5 days 23 h	(Left)	2	+	Halfway, hemorrhage
		(Right)	3	+	Halfway, hemorrhage
KT 926/27	5 days 23 h	(Left)	3	None	No
		(Right)	1	None	No
KT 928/29	5 days 23 h	(Left)	1	+	Halfway, hemorrhage
		(Right)	3	+	Halfway, hemorrhage
KT 723	6 days 3 h	Total	6	+	Halfway, hemorrhage
KT 919	6 days 3 h	(Left)	4	+	More than half, hemorrhage
		(Right)	4	+	More than half, hemorrhage
		Two of them in resorption			

Figs. 46–51: Differentiation of egg cylinder: 5 days 23 h

FIG. 46. Drawing of uterus at 5 days 23 h.
KT 928/29

FIG. 47. Low magnification of uterus, cross section.
M = mesometrium, U = disappearing uterine lumen.
KT 914. 34:1

FIG. 48. Implantation site. The ectoplacental cone appears diffuse in its peripheral region.
Z = decaying uterine epithelium, in the original lumen. 100:1

FIG. 49. Egg cylinder, retarded in development by about 24 h.
KT 926, 5 days 23 h. 270:1

FIG. 50. Differentiation of egg cylinder.
KT 929, 5 days 23 h. 100:1

FIG. 51. Detail of Fig. 48.
Some scattered cells of the ectoplacental cone have differentiated into ectoplacental glycogen cells
(eG = dashed boundaries). Maternal blood (B), only faintly stained, fills the interspace. 270:1

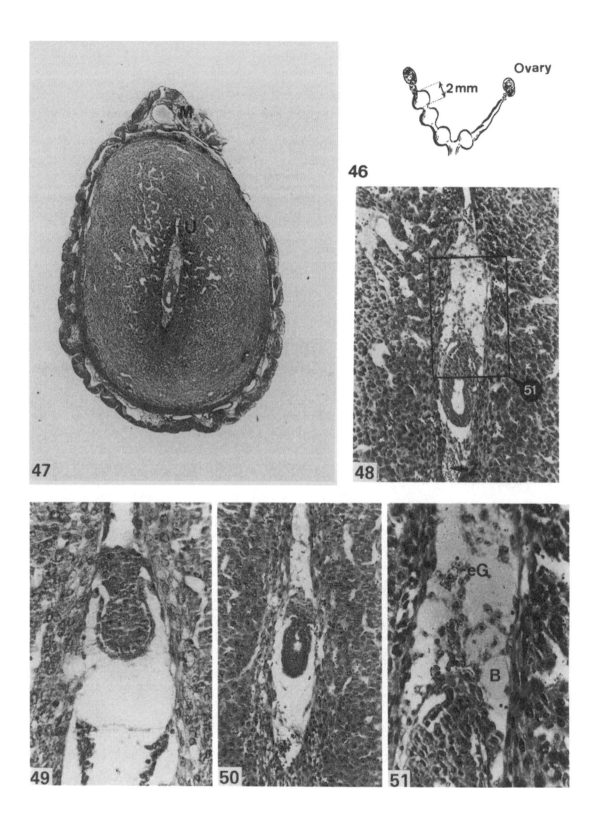

Horizon VI
Primitive villi,
distinct yolk sac.
Horizon VII
Branching villi,
axis of germ disc defined

Stage 9   Advanced Endometrial Reaction
6 1/2 Days

By 6 1/2 days, the structure of the uterine mucosa is not much different from what it was on the 6th day. By 7 days, it still may not have changed, mainly because of the variation in the degree of development of specimens having the same copulation age. The uterine reaction was examined in detail in a specimen of 6 days 20 hours, which was somewhat retarded in development. The specimen is regarded as typical of 6 1/2 days. The structure of the implantation site, rather than the structure of the embryo, was chosen by Streeter [6] to define the comparable human age.

Uterine Reaction

After the disintegration of the uterine epithelium, the ectoplacental cone is invaded by blood (Fig. 51). The original lumen of the uterine crypt has disappeared. In this way, the developing placenta gains a solid contact with its environment and with the mesometrial blood vessels. The *deciduous cells* are manifold in appearance (Fig. 55). Deciduous glycogen cells with coarse droplets are seen near the periphery of the deciduous transformation zone, predominantly in the mesometrial direction. At the same time, large capillaries invade this area. Probably the capillary invasion is necessary for the rapid production of glycogen. The other deciduous cells contain only fine, diffusely distributed glycogen. Many mitoses can be found, sometimes irregular in appearance, and they resemble those in malignant tumors. This impression is enhanced by the appearance of several multinucleated giant cells (Fig. 55).

Embryonic Axis

During this stage of development, the embryonic axis is determined. A limiting furrow, *F* (Fig. 56) is situated cranially, at the front end of the embryo. Later on it deepens (Fig. 66). In the mouse, no clearly prominent primitive knot appears, and a defined primitive groove does not form until later.

Material	Age	
KT 654/55	6 days 20 h	7 egg cylinders, H.-E.

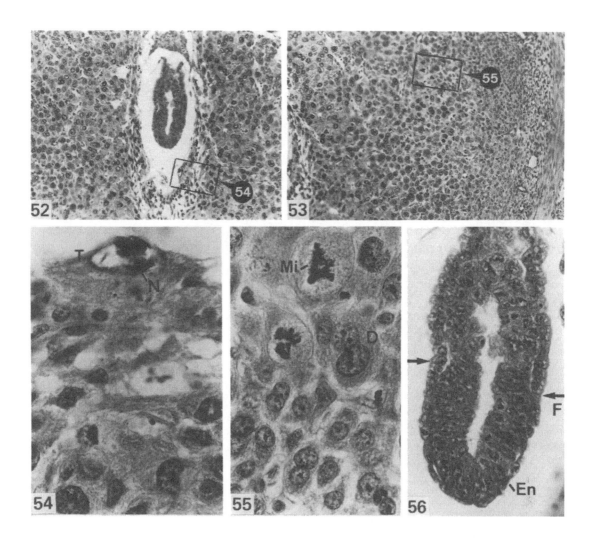

Figs. 52–56: Advanced endometrial reaction: 6 days 20 h

FIG. 52. Implantation site, low magnification.
An artificial cleft is seen between egg cylinder and ectoplacental cone.
KT 654. 100:1

FIG. 53. Deciduous boundary zone, low magnification.
KT 654. 100:1

FIG. 54. Detail of Fig. 52.
T = primary, trophoblastic giant cell with clear spherical nucleus containing a large nucleolus, *N*, and coarse chromatin, which is partially attached to the nucleolus. 700:1

FIG. 55. Detail of Fig. 53.
Boundary zone of deciduous expansion.
Irregular mitosis (*Mi*) and multinucleate deciduous cells (*D*). 700:1

FIG. 56. Egg cylinder with proamniotic cavity.
The boundary between embryonic and extraembryonic area is marked with *arrows*. *F* is the cranial limiting furrow of the embryo. The entoblastic cells become flattened at the free end of egg cylinder (*En*).
KT 654. 270:1

Stage 10   Amnion
7 Days

At 7 days, the shape of the extraembryonic part of the egg cylinder changes rapidly. A crescent-like *transverse fold* [41] temporarily appears, and pushes into the proamniotic cavity just caudal to the primitive streak. It was observed as a regularly occurring structure by Snell and Stevens [2]. It is perhaps a result of the rapid growth that occurs in the posterior wall of the egg cylinder at this time. It disappears in the following stage.

Formulation of Amnion

The tissue at the posterior end of the primitive streak bulges into the proamniotic cavity, and forms the *posterior amniotic fold*. It is continuous with the smaller lateral amniotic folds which unite to form the anterior amniotic fold. In this way, a continuous constriction forms around the middle of the egg cylinder, which is drawn tighter and tighter as the folds develop (Fig. 64). Finally, the lips of the folds will fuse and the amniotic cavity will be sealed off completely. In all embryos of this stage it is still open.

In the mesoderm of the posterior amniotic fold, small cavities appear between the cells, which coalesce to form a single large cavity, the *exocoelom*. The exocoelom is lined, except for the allantois, by a mesothelium.

Figs. 57–63: Formation of amnion: 7 days

FIG. 57. Low magnification of uterus, cross section.
U = remnant of uterine lumen, specimen between 76 and 77 days.
No extraembryonic transverse fold. 22.5:1

FIG. 58. Low magnification of uterus, cross section.
Zo = vascular zone developing. The section passes closely lateral to the connecting stalk of the egg cylinder.
KT 948, 7 days 3 h. 25:1

FIG. 59. Reconstruction, starting from a parasagittal section.
Dashed line indicates hidden lumen of egg cylinder, K = ectoplacental cone, Q = transverse fold, (*below*) the bulge of the amniotic fold.
KT 948, 7 days 3 h

FIG. 60. Egg cylinder.
KT 948, 7 days 3 h. 130:1

FIG. 61. Detail of Fig. 60.
C = lumen formation in mesoderm of the posterior amniotic fold, Q = extraembryonic transverse fold. 350:1

FIG. 62. Sagittal section through egg cylinder.
Embryo bt 76, 7 days. 90:1

FIG. 63. Detail of Fig. 62.
En = entoderm, Ek = ectoderm, M = mesoderm. 270:1

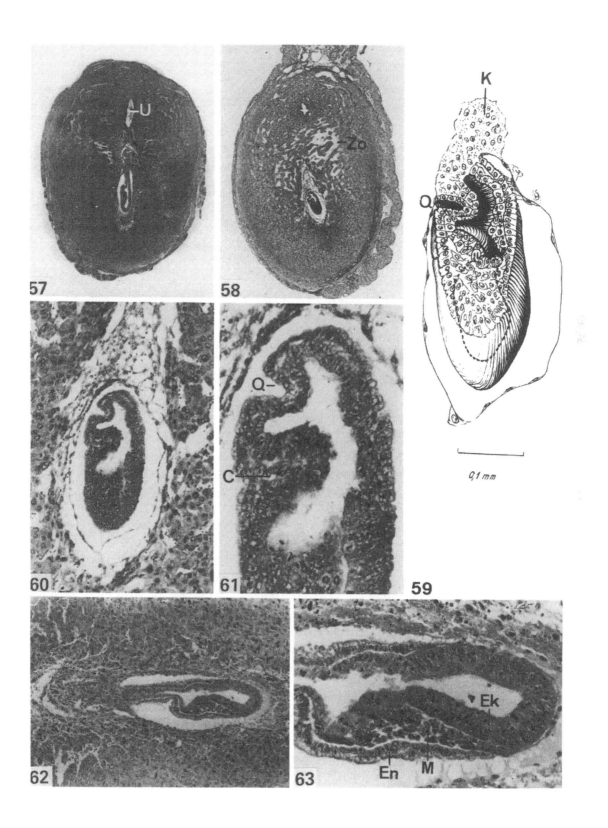

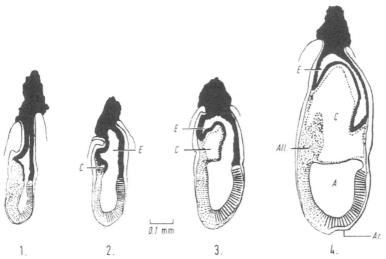

FIG. 64. Formation of amnion. (1) 7 days, (2) 7 days 3 h, (3) 7 days 10 h, (4) 7 days 20 h. The extraembryonic coelom is developing (3) by enlargement of the tiny lumina *C* (2). The coelomic mesothelium (*dashed line*) pushes between the amniotic cavity, *A*, and the ectoplacental cavity, *E*. The allantois (*All*) at first grows free into the coelom. *Black* = extraembryonic ectoderm, *Ar* = archenteron.

Formation of Mesoderm

The first mesoderm cells appear at the posterior end of the egg cylinder. As a consequence, its wall thickens and becomes three-layered (Fig. 63). In sagittal sections, the wedge-shaped head process may be observed between the flattened entoderm (*En*) and the ectoderm (*Ek*). The notochord cannot be yet identified.

Entoderm

Toward the ectoplacental cone, the cells of the visceral entoderm are cylindrical in shape and possess many vacuoles. These do not contain lipids or glycogen. However, in cryostatic sections very fine lipid droplets may be seen in the other parts of the cytoplasm. After fixation in Carnoy's solution, there is an intense PAS-reaction which is strictly limited to the superficial layer. The stained polysaccharide does not seem to be glycogen [29].

Endometrium

In the mesometrial side of the uterus, the capillaries enlarge and form distinct sinusoids (Fig. 58). The original *lumen of the uterus* is adjacent to this area , and is sometimes narrowed to a small continuous tube. The lumen becomes discontinuous in the next stage.

Material	Age	
KT 889	7 days 0 h	1 egg cylinder with extraembryonic transverse fold
KT 947/48	7 days 3 h	8 egg cylinders with extraembryonic transverse fold
		1 young egg cylinder without extraembryonic transverse fold, without mesoderm
Bt 76	7 days	1 egg cylinder without extraembryonic transverse fold, but formation of mesoderm visible

28

Stage 11   Neural Plate, Presomite Stage
7 1/2 Days

Some retarded specimens of 7 days 20 hours were included in this stage. Developmental differences between embryos of the same nominal age still exist.

Closure of Amnion

At 7 1/2 days, the amniotic cavity is sealed off. From now on, there are three separate cavities: amniotic cavity, exocoelom, and ectoplacental cleft (Figs. 64 and 72b). For a while the cleft extends as the *ectoplacental duct* to the amnion. Shortly before the development of the foregut, this duct is pushed away from the front wall of the egg cylinder by the enlarging exocoelom. It persists for awhile as a short blind extension.

The neural plate is clearly delimited anteriorly and laterally. In the midline, it forms a shallow groove. Posteriorly it is less clearly defined and merges with the primitive streak (Fig. 70). In front of the neural plate, a small oral plate consisting of two epithelia can be seen. It is just posterior to the small heart rudiment (Fig. 74).

The head process is now developing. The flattened entodermal cells situated at the free end of the egg cylinder disappear. Therefore, the head process is directly exposed to the lumen of the yolk sac. It is obviously intercalated secondarily into the entoderm and cannot be distinguished from it with certainty. In the midline, its cells become cylindrical; posteriorly they form the *notochordal plate*, which is slightly indented. This indentation has also been called the *archenteron* (Fig. 69).

The archenteron is a transitory structure that has nothing to do with the formation of the hind gut. The development of the notochordal plate is similar to the formation of the notochordal canal in the human. In mice, no canal and no distinct primitive pit exist. A "canalis neurentericus" is also completely lacking.

Foregut

At 7 days, a small furrow appears in the entoderm beneath the anterior amniotic fold (Figs. 66 and 67, *F*). It is situated at the boundary between the embryonic and extraembryonic region, *anterior* to the developing heart rudiment, in the area of what later will be the septum transversum [41]. The structure of the entodermal cells in this area changes markedly. Sometimes this change can already be seen at 6 days (in Fig. 50 this is represented by a slight constriction in the middle of the right wall of the egg cylinder). The foregut pocket will develop *caudal* to this constriction (Fig. 74).

Material	Age	
KT 996	7 days 10 h	8 egg cylinders. Formation of amnion
		1 pathologic egg cylinder, without lumen
KT 954/55	7 days 20 h	8 neurulae, presomite stages
		2 of them implanted in close proximity
KT 687	8 days 0 h	4 neurulae, presomite stages
		2 somite stages: 1 and 2 somites; deep foregut portal
		1 in resorption

Figs. 65–71: Neural plate, presomite stage, 7½ days

FIG. 65. Low magnification of uterus, cross section.
U = remnant of uterine lumen.
KT 996/2, 7 days 10 h. 24:1

FIG. 66. Detail of Fig. 65.
H = posterior amniotic fold, F = furrow in entoderm. The exocoelom (marked throughout with *)
is also visible within the anterior amniotic fold.
KT 996/2, 7 days 10 h. 270:1

FIG. 67. Tangential section of lateral amniotic fold, with exocoelom*.
Q = extraembryonic transverse fold, E = ectoplacental cavity, F = fold in entoderm.
KT 996/3, 7 days 10 h. 130:1

FIG. 68. Low magnification, slightly older stage.
M = mesometrium.
KT 954/1, 7 days 20 h. 20:1

FIG. 69. Head process with archenteron, Ar.
A = amniotic cavity, B = blood islet, E = ectoplacental cavity, * = exocoelom, K = head fold.
KT 954/1, 7 days 20 h. 100:1

FIG. 70. Detail of Fig. 68, showing allantois (All), E = ectoplacental cavity, A = amniotic cavity,
* = exocoelom, P = primitive streak.
KT 954/1, 7 days 20 h. 100:1

FIG. 71. Higher magnification of allantois (All) and Reichert's membrane (R).
E = ectoplacental cavity, * = exocoelom.
KT 954/1, 7 days 20 h. 270:1

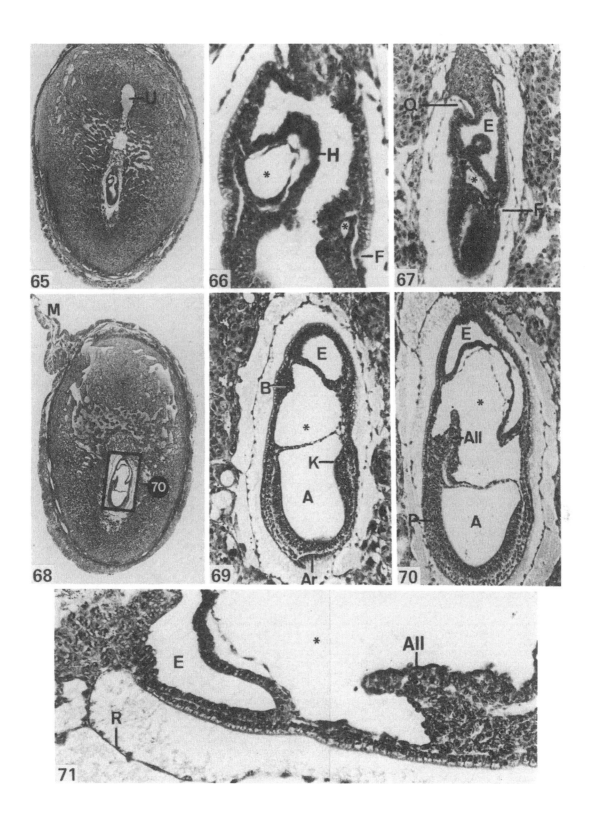

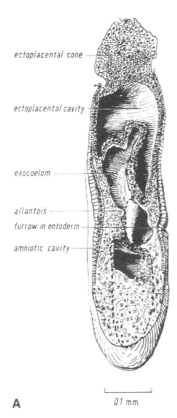

ectoplacental cone

ectoplacental cavity

exocoelom

allantois

furrow in entoderm

amniotic cavity

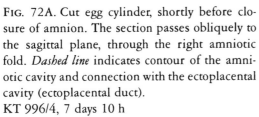

A   0.1 mm

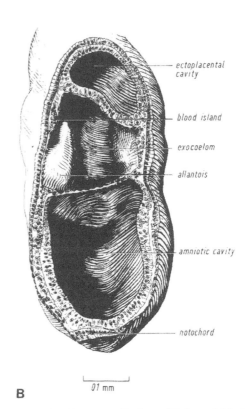

ectoplacental
cavity

blood island

exocoelom

allantois

amniotic cavity

notochord

B   0.1 mm

FIG. 72A. Cut egg cylinder, shortly before closure of amnion. The section passes obliquely to
the sagittal plane, through the right amniotic
fold. *Dashed line* indicates contour of the amniotic cavity and connection with the ectoplacental
cavity (ectoplacental duct).
KT 996/4, 7 days 10 h

FIG. 72B. Cut egg cylinder of 7 days, 20 h (after
closure of amnion).

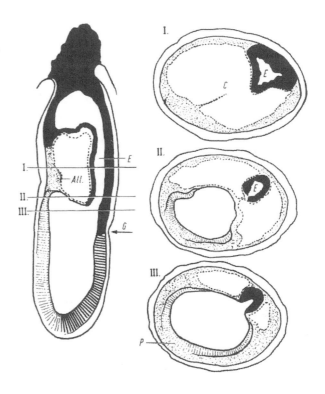

Fig. 73. Ectoplacental duct, shortly before closure of the amnion.
The drawing (*left*) shows the location of cross sections *I–III*.
E = ectoplacental duct, *P* = transition of primitive streak and extraembryonic mesoderm, *C* = mesothelial septum (in regression), *All* = allantois, *G* = limiting furrow.

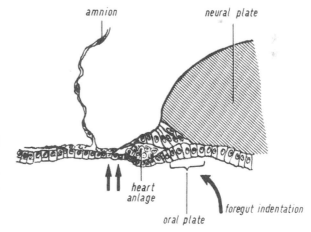

Fig. 74. Development of the foregut pocket.
Double arrow marks the embryonic–extraembryonic boundary. Here the epithelium is markedly reduced in height.
KT 955/5, 7 days 20 h

Stage 12 First Somites
8 Days, 1–7 Somites

The copulation age of this group ranges from 7 days 21 hours to 8 days 21 hours. The seven somite embryo was chosen as the most advanced in this stage because with the formation of the eighth somite, the embryo begins to rotate around its longitudinal axis. In the human, the corresponding age group, as described by Streeter [6], extends from 1 to 12 somites. The number of somites is the most reliable criterion to determine developmental age.

External Form

A conspicuous characteristic of this stage is the progressive deepening of the neural groove. There is a marked dorsal (lordotic) flexure, and rotation has not yet begun. The head fold will bulge within a few hours (Figs. 76 and 80). The *anterior intestinal portal* deepens simultaneously. The posterior intestinal portal is beginning to form. It should not be confused with the archenteron (Fig. 77).

The *allantois* has grown out far into the exocoelom toward the ectoplacental cone. In a specimen of 6 somites it was still unattached, whereas in a littermate of 7 somites (KT 639/b4) it had made firm contact with the developing chorion. Fig. 77 shows a contact already established in a 5-somite embryo. The allantois is continuous cranially with the *primitive streak*. The latter is limited anteriorly by a "quasi primitive knot," which is caused by the bulging of the underlying archenteron (Figs. 77 and 80). If the archenteron forms only a shallow groove, this prominence is not distinct (Fig. 82).

Circulatory System

Blood islets develop during the preceding stage (7 1/2 days) in the wall of the yolk sac (Fig. 69). They are arranged as a girdle encircling the exocoelom, and may be seen in each section. Fig. 83 shows the marked mitotic activity of the hemocytoblasts [46]. There is no vascular connection yet with the vessels developing in situ in the body of the embryo. The *A. vitellina* arises first as paired vascular islands in the wall of the posterior intestinal portal (Fig. 82). Later, these anlagen unite to form a single, unpaired vessel [49].

The *heart rudiment* develops rapidly as seen, for instance, in 6-somite embryos. The first visible sign is a thickening of the mesoderm surrounding, horseshoe-like, the front end of the embryo. This cellular strand can even be seen in sections of presomite stages (Fig. 74).

The pericardial cavity first develops as lateral clefts in the mesoderm. At the 2-somite stage these intercellular gaps are clearly visible on each side of the midline (Fig. 81). At the 6-somite stage a distinct lumen also appears in median sections (Fig. 82). At the same time, single mesodermal cells have joined to form an endocardial tube. This tube is continuous with the *first aortic arch*, which developed in situ along with the paired dorsal aortae.

The dorsal aorta originates bilaterally in the trunk region, beneath the somite stalks, and is visible in many cross sections (Fig. 79).

Intestinal Tract

The anlage of the foregut pouch has appeared in the preceding age group (Fig. 74). The epithelium of the gut is columnar in this area and adheres, for a short distance, to the high columnar epithelium in front of the neural plate. Both epithelial layers together form the *oral plate*. With the appearance of the first somite, the shallow groove quickly deepens to form a curved pocket (Fig. 82) narrowed ventrally by the prominent cardiac bulge. Most of the gut epithelium covering the bulge is cuboidal. The rudiment of the thyroid gland and of the liver develop here, but they cannot be distinguished yet with certainty. At the end of this period, the thyroid anlage appears as a distinct thick epithelial plate.

The notochord is situated in the dorsal wall of the foregut pocket. It is still intercalated in the entoderm, later it will become separated. It consists of a long strand of columnar cells (Fig. 78) and still has a shallow groove posteriorly (the archenteron). The gut epithelium is flattened where it joins the notochord. Anteriorly, the wide first branchial cleft forms in the foregut pocket.

At the 2-somite stage the *posterior intestinal portal* is visible as a slight depression (Fig. 80), which deepens more slowly than the anterior one. At the 6 somite stage, it is only a slight depression (Fig. 82). The lining entodermal cells are higher than other cells in the area. Further caudally, in the extraembryonic area, is the epithelium of the visceral yolk sac with its characteristic cylindrical cells with vacuolated cytoplasm and basally located nuclei (Fig. 83). The superficial layer of the cytoplasm is strongly PAS-positive. The *cloacal membrane*, in contrast to the comparable stage in human embryos, has not yet appeared.

The *coelom* originates in the trunk region within the thickened marginal band of mesoblastic cells. Vesicles appear between the mesoblastic cells, which coalesce to form a continuous mesoblastic cavity (Fig. 79). It is in open communication with the pericardiac cavity. In the older members of this group, it opens freely into the exocoelom on both sides.

Central Nervous System

In this stage, the brain plate develops very rapidly, and is the chief determiner of the embryonic form (Fig. 75). At 7 somites, the neural folds close at the level of the 4th and 5th somite, i.e., at the cervico-cranial boundary. From here, the closure proceeds both in anterior and posterior direction, in a zipper-like manner. Near the still widely open cranial end, a bilateral depression may be seen, the *optic evagination* (sulcus opticus, Fig. 75). Further caudally, two *neuromeres* [162] are visible. They are called "rhombomere *A* and *B*," homologous to the neuromeres in the human (Fig. 82). Rhombomere *B* is found at the level of the *otic placode*, which is visible at 4 or 5 somites.

In the area of the *cranial neural crest* [151] the trigeminal and facial crest are distinct.

Extraembryonic Membranes

In the preceding stage, three separate cavities were formed: amniotic cavity, exocoelom, and ectoplacental cavity (Fig. 64). During this period the exocoel and the amniotic cavity expand at the expense of the ectoplacental cavity. Toward the end of this period, both ectoplacental layers fuse in the middle (Fig. 84). Laterally, both layers (*laminae*) are still recognizable (Fig. 77). At the same time, the *allantois* grows rapidly across the exocoelom, toward the ectoplacental cone. The ectoplacental cells are delimited from the exocoelom only by a thin mesodermal lining. The first contact of the allantois is made with these cells which frequently, at the point of contact, are detached from the adjacent ectoplacental tissue. It appears as a bulge toward the approaching allantois (Fig. 80). A more laterally situated point of contact occurs rarely (for example, see Fig. 77). The time of fusion appears to vary also. It does not occur before the 5-somite stage, and is usually observed at 7–8 somites. The allantois itself transforms in its distal part into a loose meshwork of cells. Between them, endothelial-lined cavities develop, which are the forerunners of the allantoic vessels (umbilical artery and vein).

The *yolk sac* is composed primarily of two layers, the thin parietal (distal) and the thick visceral (proximal) entoderm. As described previously, only the vascular area of the visceral layer develops into the yolk sac proper. It enlarges now considerably. In later stages, this membrane can easily be recognized when the uterus is dissected. It is the inner lining of the narrow yolk sac cavity. Externally, the cavity is bound by the thin parietal layer and *Reichert's membrane* (Fig. 71). Adherent to Reichert's membrane is a layer of *trophoblastic giant cells*, which grows rapidly in thickness, and finally forms a loose network of cells (Fig. 84, indicated by *small circles*). This area attaches the embryonic to the maternal tissue.

The adjoining *endometrium* has some multinucleate giant cells, already seen in the previous stage (Fig. 55). The decidua capsularis contains only a few blood vessels, whereas the decidua basalis has large sinusoids.

In the *ectoplacental cone* a special zone of glycogen-containing cells [29] becomes visible after PAS-staining (Fig. 84, *eG*). The cells are also seen in the preceding stage, but they were less numerous (Fig. 51, 6 days). With H.-E.-staining, they are inconspicuous; however, they can be recognized by their numerous vacuoles in the faintly staining cytoplasm. Abundant storage of glycogen is characteristic of the cone cells, which are differentiating into trophospongium (junctional zone) [38].

Figs. 75–81: First somites, 8 days

FIG. 75. Dorsal view of 7-somite embryo.
Arrow marks the optic sulcus, *So5* = somite 5. 63:1

FIG. 76. Low magnification of uterus, cross section.
M = mesometrium.
KT 957/4, 7 days 21 h, 5 somites. 18:1

FIG. 77. Detail of Fig. 76.
All = allantois, *Ar* = archenteron, *P* = primitive streak, *V* = foregut pocket. 54:1

FIG. 78. Cross section posterior to the second somite.
Beginning of somite formation, *Ch* = notochordal plate.
KT 984/3, 2 somites. 270:1

FIG. 79. Cross section through the 5th somite, narrowest region of the neural groove.
Ch = notochord, *Ao* = dorsal aorta, *So 5* = somite 5.
KT 939/b5, 7 somites, 8 days 1 h. 560:1

FIG. 80. Low magnification of uterus, cross section, containing 2-somite embryo, cut longitudinally.
U = remnant of uterine lumen.
KT 984/2, 8 days 4 h. 22:1

FIG. 81. Detail of Fig. 80 with front end of embryo.
Arrow in foregut pocket, *He* = heart rudiment, *Ra* = oral plate. 560:1

36

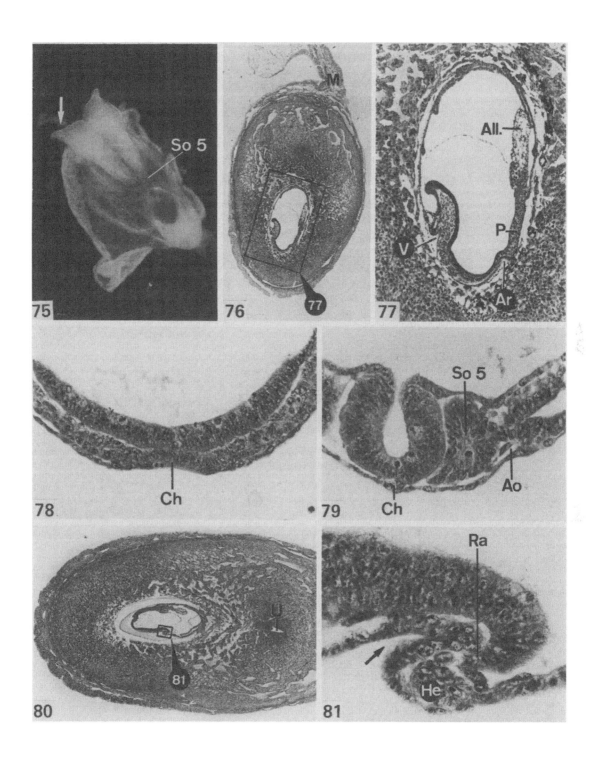

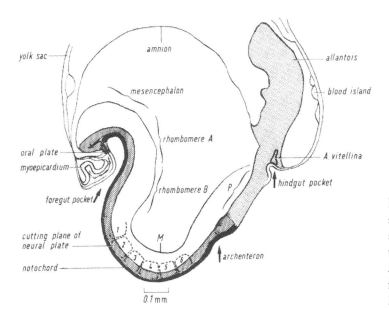

FIG. 82. Reconstruction of specimen, 8 days 1 h, 6 somites (numbered), in sagittal plane.
M = contour of right neural fold, P = primitive streak.
KT 639/b 15

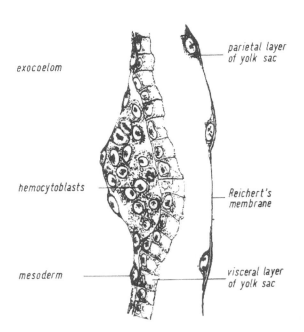

FIG. 83. Blood islet at 7 days 21 h, 5 somites.
Numerous mitoses.
KT 957/4

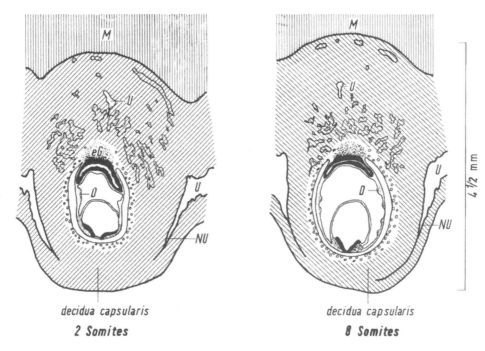

decidua capsularis
2 Somites

decidua capsularis
8 Somites

4 ½ mm

FIG. 84. Endometrium and embryonic membranes.
Maternal tissue shaded, *M* = mesometrium, *U* = old uterine lumen. The new lumen, *NU*, advances toward the antimesometrial pole, *eG* = ectoplacental glycogen cells. *Circles* = trophoblastic giant cells. Enlargement of the vascularized yolk sac (*D*). Ectoplacental cavity disappears.

Material	Age	
KT 956/57	7 days 21 h	2 with 5 somites
		5 with 5–8 somites
		1 resorption
KT 639	8 days 1 h	6 with 5–9 somites
KT 880/81	8 days 1 h	7 early somite stages (5 somites)
KT 983/84	8 days 4 h	1 presomite neurula
		2 with 1 somite
		1 with 2 somites
		2 with 3 somites
		2 with 4 somites
KT 958/59	8 days 4 h	2 presomite neurulae
		4 with 4–6 somites
		3 resorptions
KT 637	8 days 21 h	3 with 4–5 somites

Stage 13 Turning of the Embryo
8 1/2 Days, 8–12 Somites

This is a relatively short period. The copulation age of these specimens still varies considerably. It extends from 8 days 1 hour to 9 days.

The rotation of the embryo results in a marked change of the external shape (Fig. 94). The highly lordotic curvature of the trunk turns into a strong dorsal, kyphotic bend. A primary lordotic curvature also exists in human embryos, but the kyphotic change is less conspicuous and does not involve a rotation. It is appropriate, therefore, to consider this period in the mouse development separately.

The *turning*: at 8 somites, the beginning of rotation can be seen in cross sections. It is first confined to the head and tail folds. The mid-trunk region remains initially in its original position, being apparently firmly attached to the yolk sac. In Fig. 95, the torsion of the posterior end with its primitive streak with respect to the mid-trunk region is apparent. Viewed from the cranial toward the caudal end, the rotation proceeds clockwise along the body axis.

Figs. 85–93: 8 somites, 8 days 21 h

FIG. 85. Reconstruction of embryo, 8 days 21 h, 8 somites.
Level of cross sections Figs. 88–92 is indicated.
KT 985

FIG. 86. Ovary with 2 corpora lutea of the same pregnancy.
Cl = corpus luteum.
KT 985. 16:1

FIG. 87. Cellular detail: 130:1

FIG. 88. Anlage of the forebrain.
Arrow indicates sulcus opticus. 180:1

FIG. 89. Anlage of the heart.
End = endocardiac vesicle, *Tr* = aortic sac, *Th* = plate of the thyreoidea. 130:1

FIG. 90. Foregut pocket (*V*).
S.v. = sinus venosus (paired), *O* = otic plate (posterior margin). 130:1

FIG. 91. Section through 1st somite (*So 1*).
V.v. = Vitelline vein. 130:1

FIG. 92. Section through 4th somite (*So 4*).
Ao = aorta dorsalis, *Pt* = peritoneal funnel. 270:1

FIG. 93. Section through primitive streak (*P*).
H = hind gut, *Au* = umbilical artery. 270:1

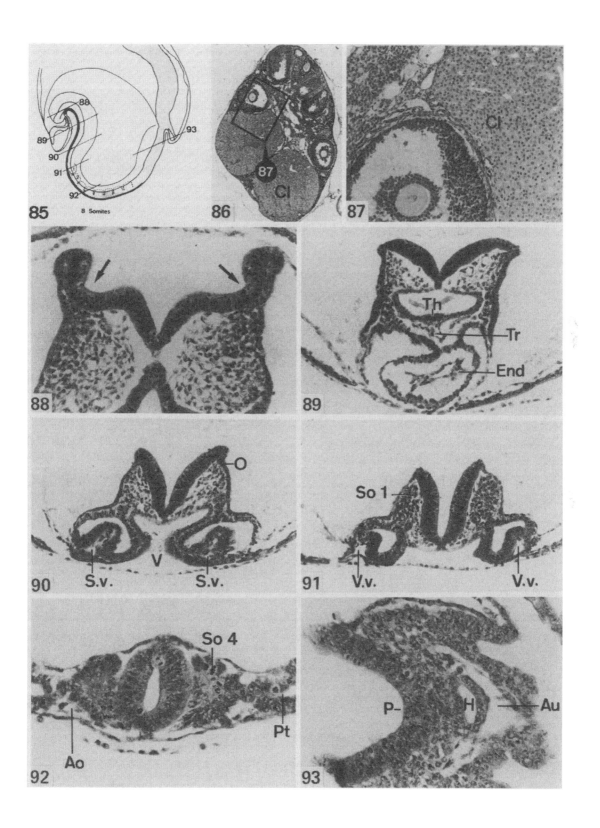

41

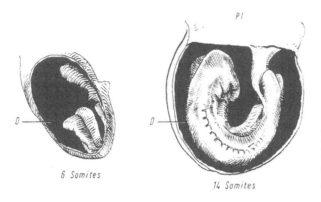

6 Somites

14 Somites

FIG. 94. Turning of the embryo. Drawing before (*left*) and after (*right*) rotation. Amnion is not shown. *D* = yolk sac (cut), *Pl* = placenta.

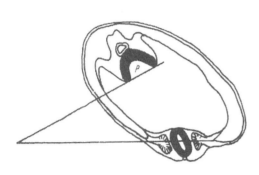

FIG. 95. Beginning rotation, 8 somites. *P* = tangential line connecting the primitive folds, shows the turning compared to the trunk.

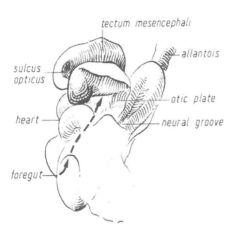

tectum mesencephali

sulcus opticus

allantois

otic plate

heart

neural groove

foregut

FIG. 96. Folding of the brain bulges. Oblique view.
Arrow indicates localization of the foregut.
KT 1002, 9 somites, 8 days 10 h

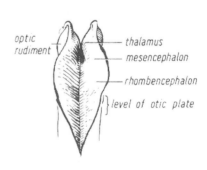

optic rudiment

thalamus

mesencephalon

rhombencephalon

level of otic plate

FIG. 97. Dorsal view of the brain folds.
They have approached each other closer in the forebrain than in the hindbrain.
KT 1002, 9 somites

42

Organogenesis

Compared to the preceding period, no radical changes occur during this stage. The previously described organ rudiments may easily be recognized, and are represented in a series of cross sections of an embryo of 8 somites (Figs. 85–93). The optic evagination is deeper now and the otic plate more distinct (Fig. 96). The thyroid rudiment [144] is clearly delimited (Fig. 89). In sagittal sections, it appears as an indentation of the foregut wall above the heart rudiment (Fig. 85).

At the end of this period, the second branchial pouch is forming. At 8 somites the first pouch is considerably enlarged, so that the entoderm contacts the overlying ectoderm. The section in Fig. 89 is immediately anterior to the contact area. The fore- and hindgut pockets are deeper now, and in the region of the somite stalks, the peritoneal funnels of the pronephros are sometimes visible (Fig. 92).

The Corpus Luteum

The structure of the corpus luteum is practically unaltered; there is little change, even when compared with the 5-day-stage (Fig. 36). The central scar and hemorrhagic traces have almost disappeared. Sometimes, a zone of loosely arranged cells is observed in this area. The histologic picture of the corpus luteum and of the interstitial gland is still unchanged.

Material	Age	Embryos
KT 639	8 days 1 h	6 with 5–9 somites (mentioned previously)
KT 1001–03	8 days 10 h	2 with 7 somites
		2 with 8 somites
		1 with 9 somites
		2 resorptions
KT 985–87	8 days 21 h	7 with 8–16 somites

Stage 14 Formation and Closure of Anterior Neuropore

9 Days, 13–20 Somites

Horizon XI
13–20 paired somites

This period could be extended to 22 somites, because the most advanced embryo, with a copulation age of 9 days 2 hours, had 23–24 pairs of somites. In the mouse, the formation of a new somite pair requires 1–2 hours. I have chosen an upper limit of 20 somites for this stage so that it will correspond to Streeter's horizon XI.

External Form

The turning of the embryo is now complete. Compared to human embryos, the mouse embryos of this group are strongly flexed in a dorsally convex direction (Figs. 99 and 108). Furthermore, there is a definite spiral torsion, the posterior end lying on the right side of the head. In rare cases, it may be found on the left side.

The external form is determined in this phase basically by the shape of the neural tube. Anteriorly, the medullary plate is about to close, whereas it is still a flat groove posteriorly. The first two branchial bars are clearly visible. The forelimb bud is not yet clearly delimited. At 15 somites, it appears as a condensation of the lateral plate material, without distinct boundaries (Fig. 100).

Length. The overall length varies considerably, mainly because of varying curvature of the body. If the amnion is cut, the embryo straightens a little. The length is measured from the crown to the curved posterior end in a straight line, and it varies from 1.2–2.5 mm. Externally, the roundish swellings of the uterus measure 3–5 mm. The spaces between the embryos are irregular in vivo, and if the mouse is killed, they are reduced by contraction of the uterus [26].

Circulatory System

In transparent fresh or formalin-fixed embryos, several vessels may be recognized by simple inspection (Fig. 108).

The broad *anterior cardinal vein* receives its blood from the close-meshed network of capillaries investing the neural tube (plexus perineuralis). It joins the posterior cardinal vein to form the *Ductus Cuvieri*.

The (paired) dorsal aorta may be seen immediately ventral to the row of somites. The endocardial tube of the bulbus cordis is very narrow and is separated by a considerable gap from the thick myoepicardium. Anteriorly it forms a right angle with the arterial trunk which is dilated at its end (aortic sac).

Development of the heart. The heart is now capable of maintaining some circulation of the blood. The atrium and ventricle are not yet paired. The shape of the arterial and venous parts of the heart, together with the connecting vessels, are shown in Figs. 109 and 110.

Placental circulation is just being established. The blood already circulates in the yolk sac. The paired dorsal aortae supply the yolk sac by means of a thick vitelline artery (Fig. 111).

This artery will originate later separately from the aorta by a new anastomosis [49], whereas the umbilical artery will remain in direct continuation of the aorta. This transformation is illustrated in Fig. 112.

Intestinal Tract

The original wide opening of the gut into the yolk sac is narrowed to a long, slender *vitelline duct*. As a consequence, fore- and hindgut are no longer represented by separate pockets, but form a continuous tube with blind ends. In the middle, it still opens into the yolk sac.

At 16 somites, the *oral plate* may rupture. At 21 somites only remnants of the membrane remain. The *cloacal membrane*, on the other hand, does not appear as a distinct membrane until the 16-somite stage, and it persists for a long time.

The *foregut* is now differentiating rapidly. The first two branchial clefts have formed (Fig. 113).

The floor of the foregut is thickened, while the dorsal epithelium remains thin. Ventrally, the *thyroid rudiment* evaginates, forming a small groove (Fig. 104). It lies just above the dilated aortic sac. Toward the end of this period, the *lung anlage* (rudiments of larynx-trachea-bronchi) appears as a ventral thickening of the epithelium. There is only a short distance between the lung rudiment and the hepatic diverticulum. This liver primordium develops earlier in mice than in humans and rapidly deepens. The stomach has not yet formed.

The coelom is a single cavity, the cavum pleuro-pericardiaco-peritoneale. In the vicinity of the umbilical ring it communicates with the exocoelom. The coelomic epithelium is thickened above the lung rudiments and in the region of the future stomach [83].

Urogenital System

In this period the somite stalks of the lower cervical and upper thoracic regions are composed of:

1. peritoneal funnel,
2. nephric vesicle; sometimes its lumen is still lacking,
3. nephric duct, as a rule still solid (Fig. 102).

At 15 somites, this typical organization can be observed at the level of the 10th to the 14th somite (KT 987). In another specimen, KT 986, with 16 somites, the pronephric duct has developed a distinct lumen at the level of the 15th somite. The anterior somites, however, are connected to the coelomic epithelium only by disorganized clusters of cells.

Germ cells [103] can be recognized in H.-E. sections for the first time at 15 somites, within the epithelium of the hind gut (KT 987).

Central Nervous System

The formation and closure of the anterior *neuropore* is a most remarkable event. It is accomplished at the same developmental phase as in humans, but seems to be displaced caudally. A comparison of Fig. 75 (7 somites) and 96 (9 somites) reveals an irregular closure of the brain folds. Initially, at 7 somites, they approach each other only posteriorly. Later, they also approach each anteriorly in the forebrain region, while there is still a wide gap in the

Figs. 98–107: Closure of anterior neuropore, 9 days, 15 and 21 somites

FIG. 98. Embryo in yolk sac (*D*) and amnion (*A*).
KT 988, 15 somites, 8 days 21 h. 7:1

FIG. 99. Dissection of embryo from membranes.
O = otic invagination.
KT 988, 15 somites. 11.5:1

FIG. 100. Oblique view of same embryo, showing anterior neuropore (*V.N.*).
Aa = forelimb. 10.5:1

FIG. 101. Cross section through embryo, 8 days 21 h, 15 somites.
Ao = aorta, *Au* = umbilical artery, *H* = hindgut.
KT 987/1. 180:1

FIG. 102. Detail of Fig. 101, with somite 14.
Ao = aorta; *Vn* = pronephric duct, without lumen here; *Pt* = peritoneal funnel. 350:1

FIG. 103. Cross section through same embryo, 15 somites, at the level of the facial nerve (*N.VII*).
V.c. = vena capitis lateralis, *Ao* = aorta, *V* = foregut.
KT 987/1. 130:1

FIG. 104. Detail of thyreoidea-anlage (*Th*).
Tr = truncus arteriosus (aortic sac).

FIG. 105. Detail of Fig. 106, showing boundary zone of ectoplacental cone.
D = yolk sac, *R* = Reichert's membrane, *T* = trophoblastic giant cells, *All* = allantois. Zone of contact with embryonic vessels, *eG* = ectoplacental glycogen cells, *De* = decidua basalis. 100:1

FIG. 106. Cross section through uterus, with embryo and extraembryonic membranes.
A = amnion, *Au* = umbilical artery in umbilical cord.
KT 624, 9 days, 21 somites. 18:1

FIG. 107. Detail of Fig. 106, showing decidua capsularis and new uterine lumen (*below*).
T = trophoblastic giant cells, forming meshwork; *R* = Reichert's membrane and distal (parietal) layer of yolk sac; *D* = yolk sac, proximal (visceral) layer, with blood vessels. 100:1

46

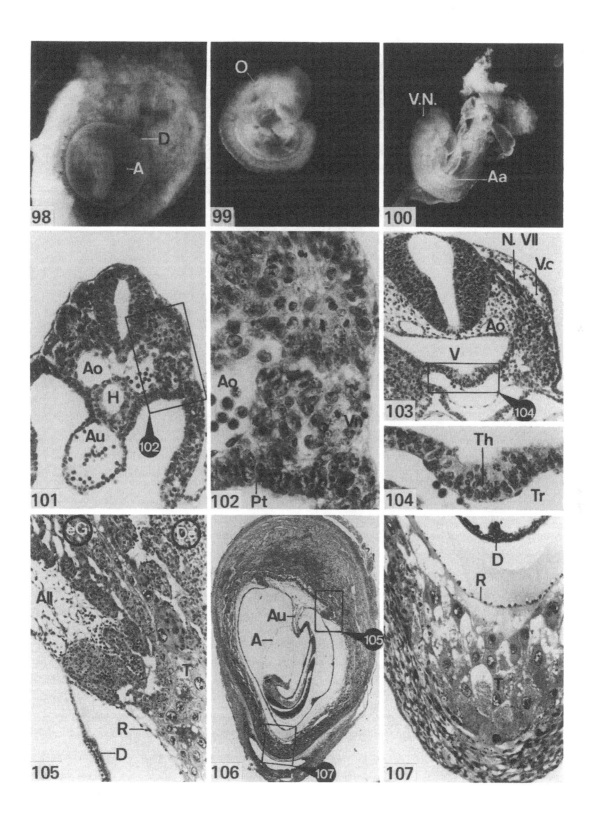

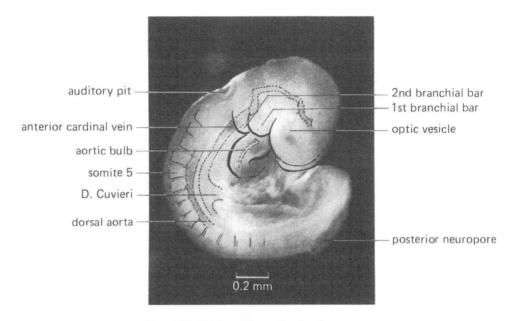

FIG. 108. Embryo, formalin fixed.
KT 937a, 14 somites, 9'days

anterior rhombencephalon (Figs. 97 and 100). They do not close in this region until 15–18 somites have formed. The closure does not coincide with the attainment of a definite somite number. The earliest was observed at 15 somites. In any case, the folds are closed at 19 somites. During dissection, a newly closed neural tube may open again, even if the uterus is fixed in toto.

After the closure of the anterior neuropore, the floor of the rhombencephalon acquires a characteristic shape. Six *rhombomeres* [162] are formed, which will disappear later. Prior to the closure of the neural tube, the rhombomeres may be seen in different phases of maturation (compare with Fig. 82).

The *cranial neural crest* [161] is visible *prior* to the closure of the brain folds. The trigeminal- and facialis crests are most distinct. In Fig. 103, the rudiment of the facialis-ganglion may be recognized. The overlying epidermis is thickened and represents the facialis-placode.

The *eye anlage* is in the vesicular stage. The optic evagination reaches the overlying epidermis prior to the closure of the neural tube and induces the formation of the lens placode. This placode can be easily recognized by the tall epithelial cells that are formed shortly after the disappearance of the anterior neuropore.

The *olfactory placode* appears shortly before the lens placode, as a striking thickening of the epithelium, while the brain tube is still open. At first it is adjacent to the forebrain. Now it begins to be separated from it by invading mesenchyme.

The *otic plate* is transforming into a deep open groove. The invagination proceeds more or less regularly with increasing somite numbers.

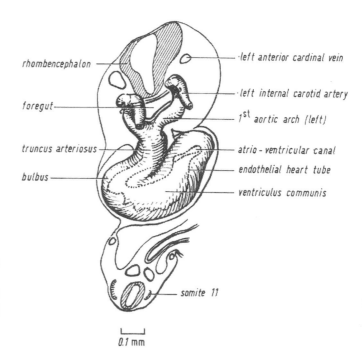

rhombencephalon

foregut

truncus arteriosus

bulbus

·left anterior cardinal vein

·left internal carotid artery

1st aortic arch (left)

atrio - ventricular canal

endothelial heart tube

ventriculus communis

somite 11

0.1 mm

FIG. 109. Reconstruction of the arterial region of the heart.
Ventral view, based on a frontal section through somite 11 and anterior rhombencephalon.
KT 987, 16 somites, 8 days 21 h

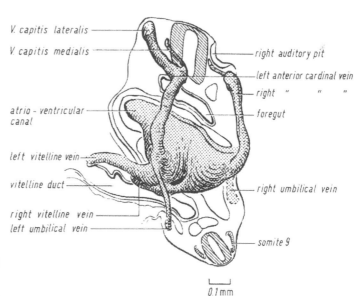

V. capitis lateralis

V. capitis medialis

atrio - ventricular canal

left vitelline vein

vitelline duct

right vitelline vein

left umbilical vein

right auditory pit

left anterior cardinal vein

right   "   "   "

foregut

right umbilical vein

somite 9

0.1 mm

FIG. 110. Reconstruction of the venous sinus.
Dorsal view, from left side. Based on a frontal section, level of somite 9 and otic invagination. The venus sinus lies dorsal to this plane.
KT 987, 16 somites, 8 days 21 h

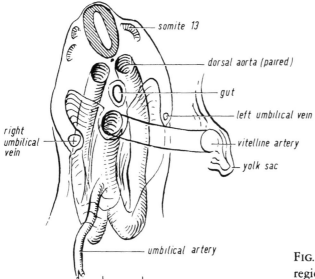

FIG. 111. Vessels of the posterior body region.
KT 987, 16 somites, 8 days 21 h

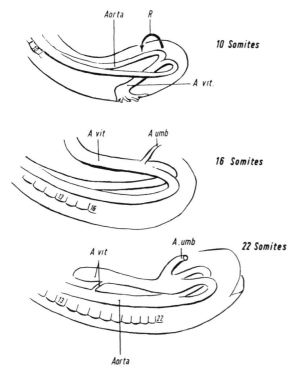

FIG. 112. Development of the posterior arterial stems. At 22 somites, the vitelline artery takes a new origin, by means of an anastomosis. The connection with the umbilical artery is lost later. The *arrow* (R) indicates the direction of the embryonic rotation.

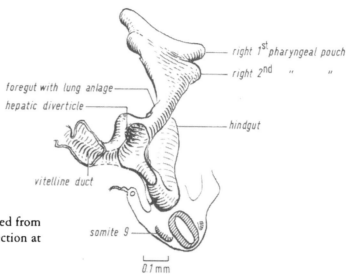

FIG. 113. Anlage of the gut, viewed from dorsal and left, starting from a section at the level of the 9th somite. 8 days 21 h, 16 somites

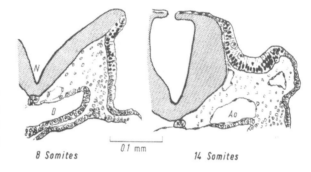

FIG. 114. Development of the otic invagination. Cross sections. The neural tube remains open here for a longer time than in human embryos. D = gut-anlage, Ao = aorta, N = neural groove.

Endometrium and Placenta

The new uterine lumen (Fig. 84) is now continuous (Fig. 106). The adjacent decidua capsularis is poorly vascularized and is composed of relatively small cells. It borders a zone of trophoblastic cells that form a perivitelline meshwork invaded by maternal blood (Fig. 107). Near this zone, the deciduous cells are often multinucleate and are darkly stained.

The *placenta* is developing in the region where the allantois reaches the ectoplacental plate ("chorionic plate"). The ectoplacental cavity disappears by fusion of the two ectoplacental laminae. The fusion begins in the middle and reaches the margins by 8 days (Fig. 77). Toward the maternal tissue, the boundary zone is organized into two different regions:

1. Toward the embryo, there is a rather solid wall of cells, into which the large allantoic vessels enter. They contain some nucleated embryonic erythrocytes (Fig. 105).
   Toward the decidua numerous clefts are developing so that the cell mass is split into anastomosing strands. The clefts are filled with maternal blood. In this way, the *labyrinth* of the placenta is formed.
2. Further toward the decidua basalis there is a zone of ectoplacental glycogen cells that are joined, more peripherally, by single trophoblastic giant cells, in continuation of the peri-

vitelline meshwork (Fig. 105). In contrast to the placental labyrinth, only *maternal blood* is circulating in this junctional zone [38] (trophospongium or reticular zone).

The yolk sac is provided now with a well formed vascular net, and it functions as additional "placenta" (yolk-sac placenta). In the course of dissection, the visceral layer of the yolk sac is immediately exposed after cutting the uterine muscular wall and decidua. There is a cleft between the proximal and distal layer, and the distal layer adheres to the decidua.

Material	Age	Embryos
KT 624–26	9 days	1 with 5 somites
		1 with 11 somites
		1 with 16 somites
		2 with 20 somites
		1 with 21 somites
		1 resorption
KT 985–88	8 days 21 h	1 with 8 somites, anterior neuropore open
		1 with 13 somites, anterior neuropore open
		2 with 14 somites, anterior neuropore open
		1 with 15 somites, anterior neuropore open
		2 with 16 somites, anterior neuropore open
		1 resorption
KT 935–37	9 days 3 h	1 with 15 somites
		2 with 17 somites, anterior neuropore closed
		1 with 20 somites, anterior neuropore closed
		3 with 22 somites, anterior neuropore closed
		1 with 23 somites, anterior neuropore closed
		1 with 24 somites, anterior neuropore closed

Stage 15 Formation of Posterior Neuropore; Forelimb Bud

9 1/2 Days, 21–29 Somites, 1.8–3.3 mm

External Shape

During this phase, the condensation of the *forelimb bud* may become apparent for the first time. It is situated at the level of the 8th–12th somite (Fig. 116). A distinct condensation of the hind limb bud does not appear until the end of this period.

A prominent feature is the presence of *3 branchial bars* compared to two in the preceding age group.

The *optic vesicle* is still spherical and has not yet begun to invaginate. In Figs. 115–116, the central light spot represents the wide open stalk of the optic vesicle and not the lens rudiment.

The *otic vesicle* is usually closed, in any case from the 24-somite stage onward.

The anterior *neuropore* is invariably closed, while the posterior one is open in all specimens examined. Compared to humans the closing of the posterior neuropore is thus retarded in mice and does not start before the next period.

Length. The extent of curvature of the embryo varies considerably, and therefore the length varies. In the fresh state, they range from 1.8 to 3.3 mm. After fixation in formalin, followed by storage in 70% alcohol, length is reduced by nearly one-third.

Sagittal Section (Fig. 121)

Figure 121 shows the relationships between some of the internal organs. Rathke's pouch is still open. The liver anlage is still covered by the heart.

Circulatory System

The *heart* consists of a convoluted tube, not yet divided into right and left parts. Through its transparent myocardial wall, the fine endocardial tube may be recognized (Fig. 118). The cardiac gelatinous coat (subendocardial jelly) contains only a few cells and is in the process of forming the atrio-ventricular cushions (Fig. 122).

The first *aortic arch* is of small caliber. The second and third are well developed (Fig. 122). They conduct the blood into the paired dorsal aortae and through the umbilical artery into the placenta. The vitelline artery (A. omphalo-mesenterica) develops a new origin from the dorsal aorta by way of a newly developed anastomosis [49] (Fig. 112).

The sinus venosus receives the same tributaries as in the previous stage (Fig. 110). However, it gradually separates from the atrium proper (atrium commune) by the development of a transverse ridge (Fig. 122).

Intestinal Tract

The intestinal tract is now undergoing important transformations, which are shown in Fig. 123.

The *lung rudiments* appear at the beginning of this period as epithelial thickenings which are now delimited posteriorly. The laryngo-tracheal groove deepens and begins to detach from the intestinal canal.

The *stomach primordium* is expanding rapidly. At the same time the omental bursa develops as a lateral peritoneal pocket (Fig. 124).

Within the *hepato-duodenal field*, columns of cells (hepatic epithelial cords) continue to invade the mesenchymal tissue of the septum transversum.

The *pancreas* develops from two separate areas of the duodenal epithelium. The anlage of the ventral pancreas is a small, circumscribed ventral evagination in the caudal part of the hepato-duodenal field. The dorsal pancreas, on the other hand, is a broad evagination in the dorsal half of the duodenal epithelium, which is not constricted until the end of this period (Fig. 123). It is not situated cranially to the ventral rudiment as in man. The reconstruction of the 10 1/2 day stage (Fig. 123) does not show the entire intestinal tract because of a lateral curvature of the embryo.

The *vitelline duct* is now closed, and its epithelium has disappeared.

Urogenital Tract

The nephric duct has grown far into the mesonephric region (Fig. 122). As an example, in specimen KT 997/5 (25 somites), it extends from the 11th to the 25th somite and parts of it have a distinct lumen. In specimen KT 939 (28 somites), the nephric duct has reached the vicinity of the cloaca (Fig. 126).

Figs. 115–120: Foreleg bud, 9 1/2 days, 22 and 24 somites, 1.8 and 2.9 mm length

FIG. 115. Embryo of 22 somites, formalin fixed, translucent.
Rh = rhombencephalon with fourth ventricle, *O* = ear vesicle, separating from epidermis. 36:1

FIG. 116. Same embryo, surface illumination.
Ab = eye vesicle, *Aa* = forelimb bud, 1 and 2 = first and second branchial bars. 36:1

FIG. 117. Same embryo, from left, translucent.
Hn = posterior neuropore. 30:1

FIG. 118. Embryo of 24 somites, formalin fixed, on a millimeter scale.
O = ear vesicle, separating from epidermis; *Aa* = forelimb-bud; *N* = suture line of neural folds; *E* = endocardium within bulbus arteriosus; *1, 2, 3* = branchial bars 1–3. 21:1

FIG. 119. Cross section of uterus with embryo of 22 somites.
Aa = forelimb bud, *Ri* = olfactory placode, *D* = yolk sac, visceral layer. 16:1

FIG. 120. Detail of Fig. 119.
Eye vesicle with emigrating cells of the ophthalmic neural crest (*Op*). 200:1

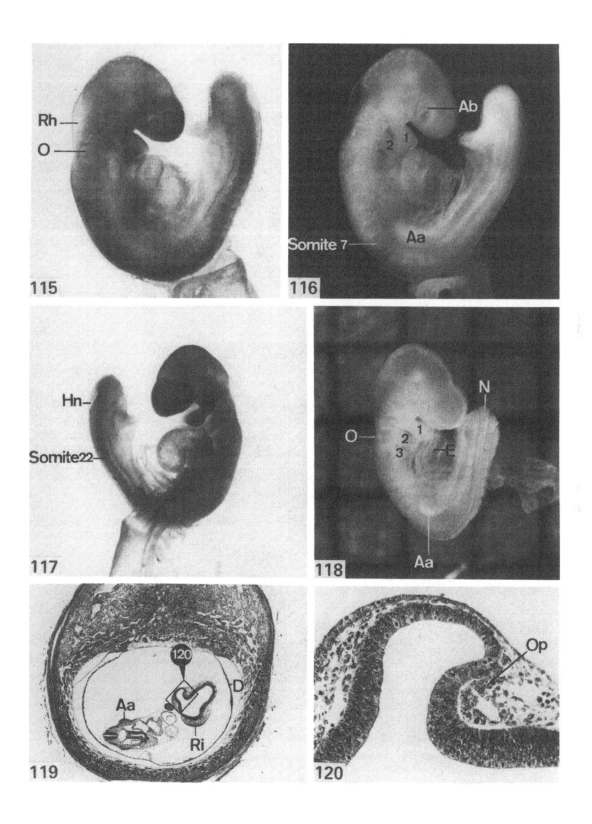

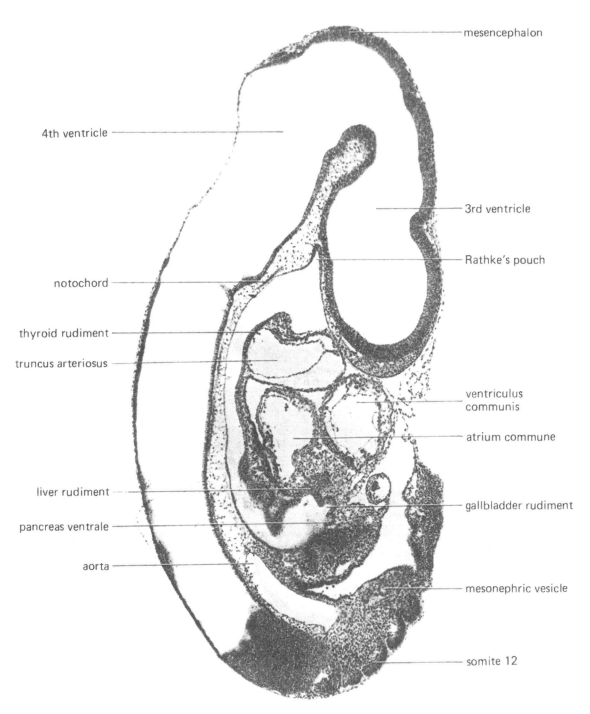

4th ventricle

mesencephalon

3rd ventricle

Rathke's pouch

notochord

thyroid rudiment

truncus arteriosus

ventriculus communis

atrium commune

liver rudiment

gallbladder rudiment

pancreas ventrale

aorta

mesonephric vesicle

somite 12

FIG. 121. Sagittal section through embryo of 10 days, 26 somites.
KT 939. 62:1

56

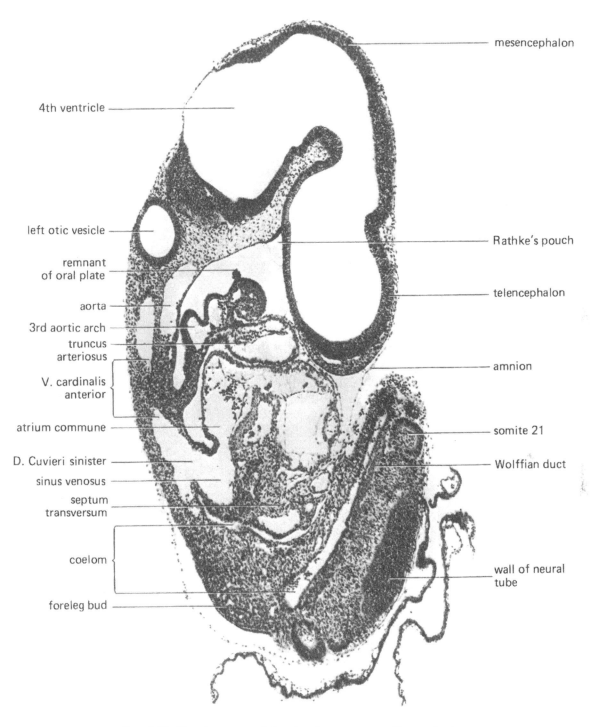

mesencephalon

4th ventricle

left otic vesicle

remnant
of oral plate

aorta

3rd aortic arch

truncus
arteriosus

V. cardinalis
anterior

atrium commune

D. Cuvieri sinister

sinus venosus

septum
transversum

coelom

foreleg bud

Rathke's pouch

telencephalon

amnion

somite 21

Wolffian duct

wall of neural
tube

FIG. 122. Development of the circulatory system. Parasagittal section through mouse embryo of 9 days 3 h.

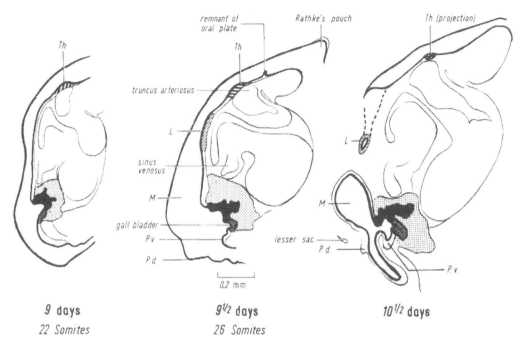

FIG. 123. Development of the intestinal tract, illustrated in 3 sagittal sections, 9–10 1/2 days, drawn to scale. *Th* = primordium of thyroid, *L* = primordium of lung, *M* = primordium of stomach, *P.d.*, *P.v.* = pancreas (dorsal, ventral); *stippled area* represents mesenchyme of septum transversum; *black area* represents liver anlage.

KT 936 9 days, KT 997 9 1/2 days, KT 999 10 1/2 days

Central Nervous System

The *posterior neuropore* begins to constrict but is still open in all embryos examined (Fig. 117), even in those with 26 or 28 somites (Fig. 126). Thus, the closure is definitely retarded in mice compared with human embryos of the same somite number. The completion of closure in mice has been observed as late as the 32-somite stage.

During this period the brain develops very rapidly. The *optic vesicles* have relatively large stalks. From the outer periphery of the vesicles, the cells of the *optic neural crest* spread into the surrounding mesenchyme (Fig. 120). They probably become pigment cells of the uvea. The other divisions of the cranial neural crest [161] have formed prior to this stage, when the anterior neuropore was still open.

The development of the cranial blood vessels parallels the extremely rapid growth of the brain. The central nervous system is being invested by an extensive vascular plexus.

The *lens placode* and the *olfactory placode* appear as distinct thickenings of the surface epithelium (Fig. 119).

The *otocyst* (ear vesicle) is completely detached from the surface at the 22–24 somite stage. It is one of the most reliable characteristics for determining the degree of development. For a while, the closing rim of the otocyst is stretched into a ductlike stalk by which the ear vesicle is attached to the surface (Fig. 125). Sometimes the process of detachment of the right and left otocyst is slightly asynchronous, but the differences observed are slight. The epithelium of the otocyst is highly specialized and is entirely different from the simple skin ectoderm. It consists of tall cells, and all mitoses are localized in the superficial layer bordering the lumen. In this respect, it resembles the wall of the neural tube.

58

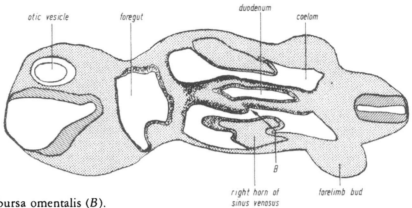

FIG. 124. Anlage of bursa omentalis (B).
KT 935/9, 9 days 3 h, 23 somites

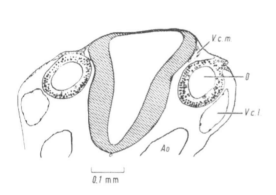

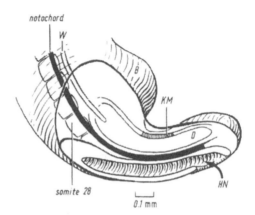

FIG. 125. Otic vesicle separating from epidermis, 9 days, 22 somites.

O = otic vesicle, *Ao* = aorta, *V.c.l.* = vena capitis lateralis, *V.c.m.* = vena capitis medialis.
KT 935

FIG. 126. Posterior part of the body. Graphic reconstruction.

10-day embryo, 28 somites; *HN* = posterior neuroporus (*arrow*); *W* = Wolffian duct; *KM* = cloacal membrane; *D* = hindgut, extending into tail bud; *B* = hindleg bud.
KT 939/3

Material	Age	
KT 935–37	9 days 3 h	4 with 15–20 somites (mentioned before)
		3 with 22 somites
		1 with 23 somites
		1 with 24 somites
KT 997–98	9 days 10 h	1 with 17 somites. Posterior neuropore open.
		1 with 22 somites. Posterior neuropore open.
		1 with 23 somites. Posterior neuropore open.
		1 with 24 somites. Posterior neuropore open.
		2 with 25 somites. Posterior neuropore open.
		2 with 26 somites. Posterior neuropore open.
KT 648–49	9 days 23 h	7 with 22–23 somites. Posterior neuropore open.
		Two of them measured 3.2 and 3.5 mm (unfixed).
KT 938–40	10 days	9 with 25–34 somites,
		Five measured 3.2–3.9 mm (unfixed).

Stage 16   Closure of Posterior Neuropore; Hind Limb Bud and Tail Bud

10 Days, 30–34 Somites, 3.1–3.9 mm (fresh)

External Shape

Some typical features of stage 16 are represented in Fig. 134. The hind limb bud becomes visible as a distinct bulge at the level of the 23rd–28th somite. The tail rudiment appears as a short stump (Fig. 127). The surfaces of the third and fourth branchial bars are distinctly concave, in contrast to the second. In this way the formation of the cervical sinus is initiated. The *lens plate* is usually slightly indented (Figs. 129–131). This corresponds to the early horizon XIV of Streeter. Lens development seems to be slightly advanced in mouse compared to human embryos. The olfactory placode is clearly indented, and is also slightly advanced in development compared to the human embryos.

The *otocyst* is invariably closed. It is no longer spherical, but more or less pear-shaped in its dorsal segment (Fig. 127).

The *posterior neuropore* begins to close.

Length. In the unfixed state, the overall length varies between 3.3 and 3.9 mm.

Circulatory System

The cardinal veins may be clearly recognized in intact embryos (Fig. 129). The heart forms a prominent bulge in the vicinity of the branchial bars. The structure of the heart is essentially the same as in stage 17 for which a detailed reconstruction is represented in Fig. 148.

Intestinal Tract

The most conspicuous change in this age group is the formation of the lung anlage (Fig. 132): the laryngo-tracheal groove branches from the esophageal gut and the two primary bronchi sprout out in a T-like manner (Figs. 132, 133). The development of the intermediate portion of the intestinal tract was shown in Fig. 123. The hindgut still has the same appearance as in Fig. 126.

Urogenital System

The nephrogenic cord is now widely separated from its origin in the somite stalks. In the pronephric region, anterior to the 12th somite, only small clusters of cells are visible, and there is no structural organization. At the level of the 12th somite, spherical groups of nephrogenic cells may be recognized. They are arranged as vesicles at the level of the 13th to the 15th somite (Fig. 135). Generally, two such vesicles will form in each segment. Maturation proceeds slowly: at the 32 somite stage, the nephrotome of the 20th somite is not much more developed than in the 26-somite stage (Fig. 135). In one 26-somite embryo, there is a peritoneal funnel. There are no mesonephric glomerula at this stage.

The *Wolffian duct* is recognizable in the younger specimen examined, and it extends from the 13th to the 26th somite. In the older specimen, it has already reached the cloaca. At the point of contact, numerous pycnotic nuclei may be seen.

Primordial germ cells [103] can be seen as large cells containing much alkaline phosphatase. Some are already situated within the genital ridge, on both sides of the dorsal mesenteric attachment.

Central Nervous System

In most cases the neural tube is now completely closed. Compared to the human embryo of similar somite number, closure is delayed in mice. As an example, specimen KT 939/4 has 32 somites, and its posterior neuropore has just closed.

The separation and differentiation of the *otic vesicle* behaves nearly exactly the same in mice as in humans. The vesicle is now closed and completely separated from the epidermis. The endolymphatic appendage is marked off as a dorsal recess from the main cavity of the vesicle, giving it a more elongated appearance.

The *olfactory placode* is considerably thickened and slightly indented.

The *ganglia* of the cranial nerves appear as distinct blastemal condensations. In transparent specimens, the large trigeminal ganglion can easily be recognized, situated just anterior to the pontine flexure of the brain tube (Fig. 127). Posteriorly, the spinal ganglia are differentiated from the neural crest.

In older specimens, the *lens plate* is slightly indented (Fig. 130).

Placenta

The loosely structured chorionic plate is traversed by the allantoic vessels. The ectoplacental plate is transformed into the labyrinth, and its margins are turned inward (Fig. 136). Consequently, the transition zone of the two yolk sac layers is also turned inward. The yolk sac cavity will later communicate here with the interplacental cavities, which develop secondarily as small clefts within the labyrinthine cell mass after disappearance of the original ectoplacental cavity [33].

The zone of "giant cells" (Fig. 136A) borders the decidua, which has many multinucleate cells in this region. Toward the mesometrium, the deciduous cells penetrate the myometrium and start to form the "metrial gland" [25].

Material	Age	
KT 938–40	10 days	4 with 25, 26, 27 and 28 somites (listed previously).
		1 with 32 somites. Posterior neuropore just closed.
		1 with 32 somites. Posterior neuropore still open.
		1 with 34 somites. Posterior neuropore closed.

Figs. 127–133:

FIG. 127. Embryo of 32 somites, from the right. Formalin fixed.
The trigeminal ganglion (*V*) is visible through the skin as well as the slightly pointed otic vesicle (*O*).
Dashed line indicates level of the section Fig. 130. 13.5:1

FIG. 128. Embryo of 30 somites, on millimeter scale. Bouin fixed.
Nominal age 11 days, developmental age 10 days.
KT 945. 13.5:1

FIG. 129. Embryo of 33 somites, from the left.
For explanations, see Fig. 134. 13.5:1

FIG. 130. Horizontal section through eye primordium, low magnification. Plane of section indicated in Fig. 127.
D = diencephalon (3rd ventricle), *Tel* = cerebral hemisphere.
KT 939/4, 32 somites. 100:1

FIG. 131. Detail of Fig. 130.
L = lens invagination, *R* = retinal sheet. 270:1

FIG. 132. Cross section, level of lung primordium. The apparent asymmetry of the lung bud is mainly due to the oblique plane of section.
V.c.a. = vena cardinalis anterior, *Ao* = aorta dorsalis (paired).
KT 939/4, 10 days, 32 somites. 100:1

FIG. 133. Detail of Fig. 132.
L = laryngo-tracheal groove. 270:1

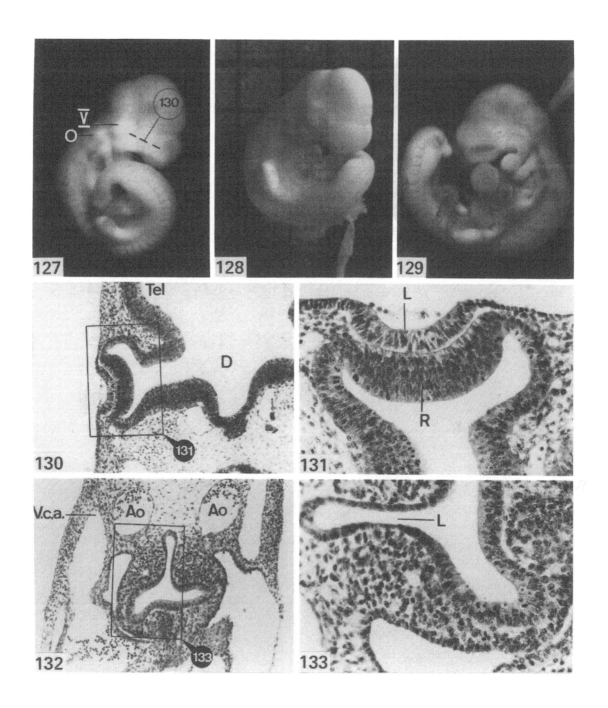

63

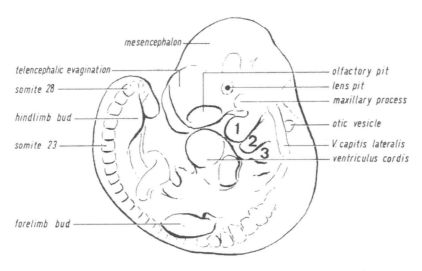

FIG. 134. Externally visible features of embryo Fig. 129, 33 somites

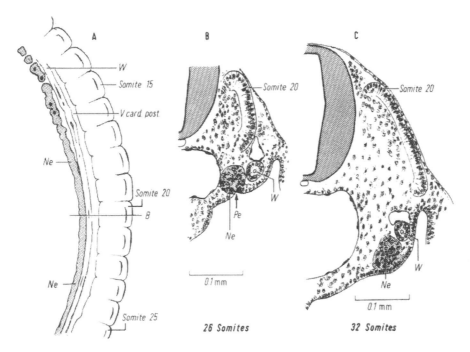

FIG. 135. Development of the mesonephros, 10 days.
(A) Drawing shows level of cross section; (B) cross section, embryo of 26 somites; (C) shows same cross section, embryo of 32 somites; *Pe* = peritoneal funnel; *Ne* = nephrogenic cord (*dotted area*); *W* = Wolffian duct.
KT 939/2

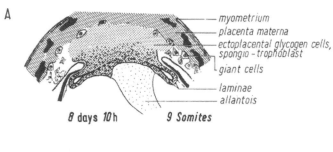

A

- myometrium
- placenta materna
- ectoplacental glycogen cells, spongio-trophoblast
- giant cells
- laminae
- allantois

8 days 10h   *9 Somites*

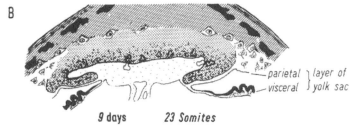

B

parietal ⎫ layer of
visceral ⎭ yolk sac

9 days   *23 Somites*

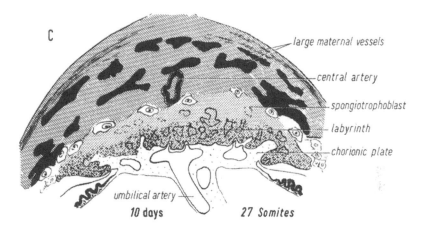

C

- large maternal vessels
- central artery
- spongiotrophoblast
- labyrinth
- chorionic plate

umbilical artery

10 days   *27 Somites*

FIG. 136. Development of the placenta.
(A) Disappearance of the ectoplacental cleft (*broken line* between laminae);
(B) margins of laminae turned inwards, (C) formation of labyrinth (*dashed area* indicates maternal tissue).
A KT 1001/4, *B* KT 935/9, *C* KT 938/4

Stage 17   Deep Lens Indentation
10 1/2 Days, 35–39 Somites, 3.5–4.9 mm (fresh)

External Shape

The *extremities* and *tail* are enlarging rapidly. They are no longer simple ridges and a short stump. Instead, they are projecting appendages and curve forward or inward. The tail is considerably longer now than in the human of this stage.

The *olfactory discs* are also more advanced, forming a distinct marginal lip. The *lens vesicles* form deep pockets (in younger embryos) or pore-like openings (older) to the surface. This is one of the best characteristics to use for assigning an embryo to this stage.

The first branchial bar is divided into large conspicuous maxillary and mandibular processes. The most cranial *somites* are becoming more and more indistinct. On the other hand, the most cranial *spinal ganglia* are easily recognized in transparent specimens. They are still completely lacking in the tail, where only somites are visible.

Behind the cloacal membrane, a short *ventral ectodermal ridge* (Grüneberg [195]) is recognizable (Fig. 146).

Length. The overall length of unfixed embryos varies from 3.5 to 4.9 mm.

Sagittal section (Fig. 145). The most prominent feature is again the advanced development of the *brain tube*. The *optic recess* (groove) is a conspicuous depression, situated just posterior to the thick commissural field and anterior to the thin optic chiasma. *Rathke's pouch* is narrowed and the median thyroid is deepened. It is shown at higher magnification in Fig. 141.

Circulatory System

With the development of the yolk sac and the placenta, two complete *extraembryonic circuits* have been established: the yolk sac and the placental circulation. The yolk sac vessels, passing along the obliterated yolk sac stalk (Fig. 137), separate distally. Only in the region close to the embryo does the vitelline vein course parallel to the vitelline artery. It separates from it distally and independently proceeds to the yolk sac (Fig. 147).

The *aorta abdominalis*, now a single unpaired vessel, forks into two branches at the level of the hind limb buds. These branches are the two umbilical arteries, and the left one is larger than the right one. The actual continuation of the original dorsal aortae is represented by two slender vessels proceeding in the dorsal body wall into the tail, nearly to its tip.

Both *umbilical arteries* unite ventral to the gut tube at the base of the umbilical ring to form an unpaired vessel.

The (unpaired) *vitelline artery* branches off from the aorta as a conspicuous vessel in the middle region of the trunk [49]. It passes cranially beside the head to the yolk sac (Fig. 147).

Both umbilical veins unite in the region of the umbilical ring by anastomoses, caudal to the umbilical and vitelline arteries. Distally, a large venous stem branches within the placenta into smaller vessels. Proximally, however, there are two asymmetrical umbilical veins which pass within the left and right body walls. The right umbilical vein is more than twice as large as the left.

The *heart* is still a single, curved tube. It has two distinct constrictions: the sulcus atrioventricularis and the sulcus sinu-atrialis (Fig. 148). The termination of the above-mentioned vitelline and umbilical veins is reconstructed in Fig. 147.

Aortic arches. The first and second arch are greatly reduced compared to the previous stage. The sixth is developing and sends a branch to the lung primordium.

Intestinal Tract

In the midline of the *pharyngeal region*, the *thyroid rudiment* is represented by a narrow diverticulum (Fig. 141). Laterally, all *pharyngeal pouches* may be seen.

The *lung bud* is rapidly elongating. The left primary bronchus is shown in Fig. 143 as a small tube.

The short *esophagus* continues into the large eccentric *stomach* anlage. This asymmetric development results in the formation of the coelomic pockets, which are conspicuous in microscopic sections (Fig. 145).

In the region of the *hepatic diverticulum*, the evaginations of the ventral pancreas and the gall bladder primordium are distinctly visible (Fig. 144). The hepatic cords are invading the mesenchyme of the septum transversum. Future erythropoietic cells seem to stem from this mesenchyme and now join these epithelial cords. The dorsal pancreas begins to constrict at its base. It grows both caudally and toward the left. In Fig. 144 (marked *P.d.*) the wall of the basal constriction is cut tangentially.

The *umbilical loop* is only slightly curved and is clearly visible in Fig. 137. The obliterated vitello-intestinal duct (yolk stalk) is attached to its apex. The vitelline vessels described previously pass through its walls to the yolk sac.

The *cloacal membrane* has not yet ruptured.

Urogenital System

The Wolffian duct has now reached the cloacal wall, where it ends blindly. The ureteric bud is forming. The mesonephric tubules are longer and more numerous than in the previous stage. However, there are no mesonephric glomeruli.

Central Nervous System

The cerebral vesicles appear as distinct bulges. The *rhombencephalic* portion of the brain is relatively large. It has an extremely thin transparent roof and a thick and wide floor with marked neuromeric elevations [162] (Fig. 143, *upper left*).

In the floor of the third ventricle, the optic recess is distinctly visible. In the *roof* of the *diencephalon*, some pycnotic cells can be regularly observed [158]. Later, at 11 or 12 days, there is a pronounced degeneration of cells [166].

The *deep lens pocket* [181] (Fig. 140), which will develop into a pore-like opening of the lens vesicle, is a characteristic of this age group.

The *otic vesicle* has developed a short endolymphatic duct (Fig. 149).

The *olfactory plate* is broad, but relatively flat, with a distinct rim (Fig. 140).

The *ganglia of the branchial nerves* are now well formed. The dorsal ganglion of the glossopharyngeal nerve is visible in Fig. 142, below the otic vesicle, close to the anterior cardinal vein (later to become the anterior jugular vein).

In the trunk region, the most anterior spinal ganglia may be seen lateral to the somites in transparent specimens.

Material	Age	
KT 909	10 days	4 embryos (all well developed), 3.3–4.4 mm.
KT 944–46	10 days 23 h	5 embryos + 1 resorption, 3.5–4.5 mm, 33–35 somites.
KT 999–1000	10 days 9 1/2 h	3 embryos + 2 resorptions, 4.0–4.5 mm.

Figs. 137–144:

FIG. 137. Embryo of approximately 36 somites.
N = umbilical loop with projecting yolk sac stalk (obliterated), 11:1

FIG. 138. Embryo, formalin fixed, nominal age 10 days, but actually further developed.
See Fig. 139 for explanation.
KT 909. 20:1

FIG. 139. Drawing of embryo (Fig. 138).
Tel = cerebral hemisphere, *L* = lens invagination, *Hl* = hindlimb bud, *Aa* = forelimb bud, *O* = otic vesicle, *Ri* = olfactory pit, *He* = heart, *So* = somite 4, C_2 = ganglion cervicale 2. Branchial bars are indicated by *1* and *2*.
KT 909

FIG. 140. Cross section through eye and olfactory pit.
L = lens pocket, *Ri* = olfactory placode, *3.V.* = 3rd ventricle.
KT 909. 100:1

FIG. 141. Thyroid primordium, sagittal section.
Th = thyroid pocket, *T.a.* = truncus arteriosus.
KT 999, 10 days 9 1/2 h 350:1

FIG. 142. Otic vesicle (*O*), oblique section (transverse-frontal).
Rh = rhombencephalon.
KT 909. 130:1

FIG. 143. Paramedian section.
Lu = lung bud (left stem bronchus), *Ao* = aorta dorsalis, *S.v.* = sinus venosus, *Coe* = coelomic pockets, * = stomach. *Arrow* indicates neural crest.
KT 999, 10 days 9 1/2 h. 40:1

FIG. 144. Detail of Fig. 142.
Lz = hepatic cell cords, *G* = anlage of gall bladder, *P.v.* = pancreas ventral, *P.d.* = pancreas dorsal (tangential section). 270:1

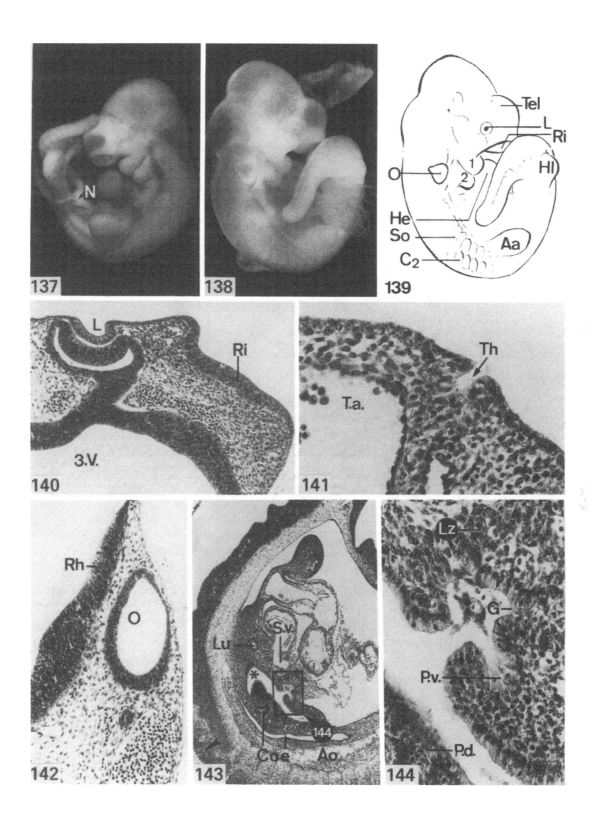

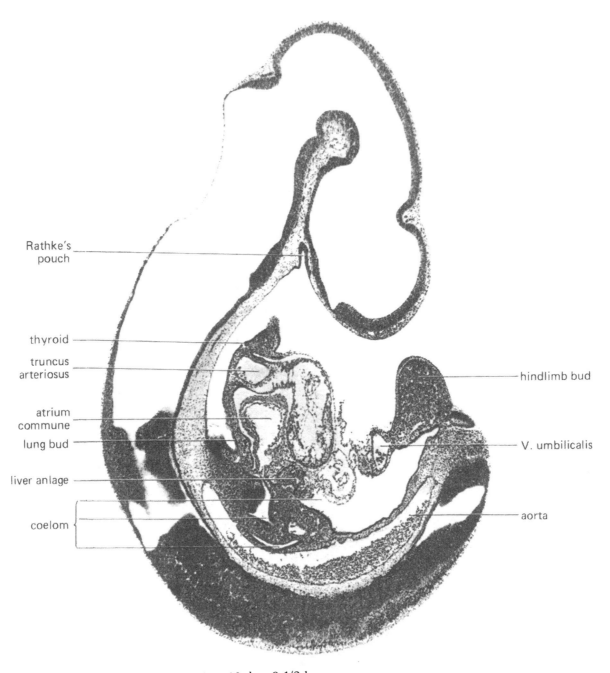

Rathke's
pouch

thyroid

truncus
arteriosus

hindlimb bud

atrium
commune

lung bud

V. umbilicalis

liver anlage

coelom {

aorta

FIG. 145. Sagittal section, 10 days 9 1/2 h.
KT 999

FIG. 146. Proximal tail in cross section.
KT 909

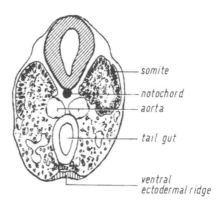

somite

notochord

aorta

tail gut

ventral
ectodermal ridge

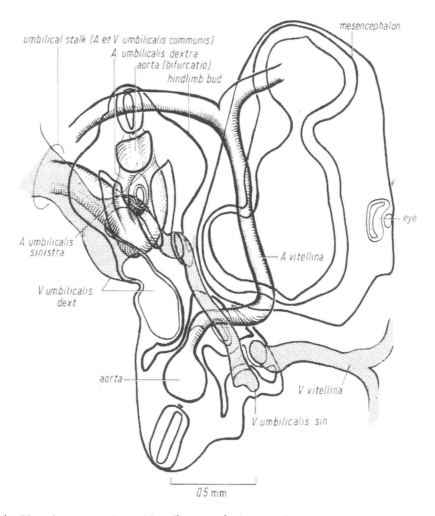

umbilical stalk (A et V umbilicalis communis)
A. umbilicalis dextra
aorta (bifurcatio)
hindlimb bud

mesencephalon

A. umbilicalis
sinistra

V. umbilicalis
dext.

eye

A. vitellina

aorta

V. vitellina

V. umbilicalis sin.

0.5 mm

FIG. 147. Vascular connection with yolk sac and placenta. Reconstruction,
starting from cross section through embryo.
KT 909

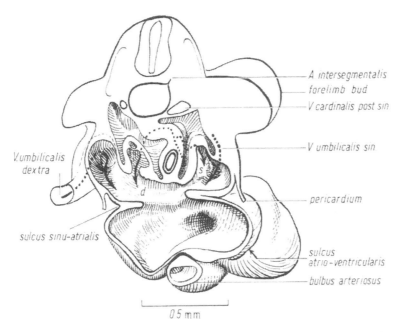

A intersegmentalis
forelimb bud
V cardinalis post sin

V umbilicalis sin

V.umbilicalis
dextra

pericardium

sulcus sinu-atrialis

sulcus
atrio-ventricularis
bulbus arteriosus

0.5 mm

FIG. 148. Sinus venosus, cross section. Reconstruction.
View from cranial: *d* = vena vitellina dextra, *s* = vena vitellina sinistra.
KT 909

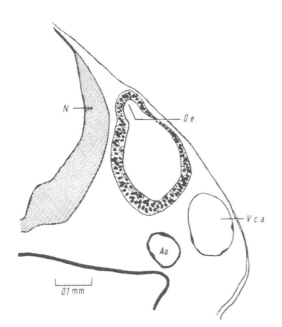

N

D.e.

V.c.a.

Ao

0.1 mm

FIG. 149. Otic vesicle with endolymphatic duct (*D.e.*).
N = neural tube (rhombencephalon), *V.c.a.* = vena cardinalis anterior, *Ao* = aorta dorsalis.
KT 909, approximately 36 somites

Horizon XIV–XV
homo = 32–33 days
6–9 mm

Stage 18   Closure of Lens Vesicle
11 Days, 40–44 Somites, 5–6 mm

External Form

The somites in the cervical region are no longer visible. They can still be recognized in the posterior part of the body, especially in the tail. The long tail passes lateral to the head, over the deep nasal pit. The external features are shown in Figs. 150–152.

Streeter did not designate a special stage to mark the closure of the lens vesicle in man. Therefore, our stage 18 is between his horizon XIV (open vesicle) and XV (closed vesicle).

Length. Unfixed embryos are 5–6 mm long.

Sagittal section. The rapid growth and maturation of the brain is striking (Fig. 158). The infundibular recess is distinct, and the opening into the lateral ventricle is beginning to form. The liver is growing rapidly.

Circulatory System

The *heart* is still a curved, undivided tube. The bulbar ridges can easily be recognized in sagittal sections (Figs. 145, 158). For the following stages (11 1/2 and 12 days), the differentiation of the bulbus arteriosus is described in more detail.

The primitive olfactory artery (arteria cerebri anterior) branches off from the *arteria carotis interna* at the same time as the nasal pits are developing.

Intestinal Tract

The *thyroid primordium* (Fig. 155) is shaped as a vesicle with a very thick basal wall. The lumen of this vesicle is a remnant of the thyro-glossal duct. It does not correspond to a thyroid follicle. In some embryos of this stage, the vesicle has separated from the surface.

The *lung bud*, stomach, and gall bladder are cut tangentially in the sagittal section shown in Fig. 158.

The epithelial lining of the dorsal mesentery of the stomach is thickened and represents the anlage of the *spleen* (Fig. 159). The thickening is part of the anterior splanchnic mesodermal plate (Green [83]).

The *cloaca* (Fig. 161) is not yet subdivided. The cloacal septum becomes evident in the next stage (Fig. 176).

Urogenital Tract

The *mesonephros* has not changed much since the preceding stage. The genital ridge is more distinct (Fig. 160), but diagnosis of the sex is not yet possible.

Central Nervous System

The brain is now more clearly subdivided, especially the diencephalon [172] with its basal recesses. The epiphyseal evagination, however, has not yet appeared. A marginal layer has formed in the brain stem (Fig. 154). The trigeminal and stato-acoustic ganglia may again be identified in transparent specimens (Fig. 152).

The *otocyst* has an elongated endolymphatic duct.

The *lens vesicle* begins to detach from the ectoderm (Fig. 153). In 2 out of 13 embryos of this group, the lumen had just lost its communication with the amniotic cavity.

The *olfactory plate* is now considerably deepened (Figs. 153 and 162). The bordering rims are beginning to unite. In the human, this stage is reached at a much later developmental phase, in horizon XVI.

Vertebral Column

Sclerotomic fissures are appearing in the trunk region. Later, they become more distinct (Fig. 186).

Material	Age	
KT 949–51	11 days 5 h	8 embryos, 4.8–5.1 mm length. 5–7 tail-somites.
KT 604–5	11 days	6 embryos, 5.0–6.2 mm length.

FIG. 150. Embryo of 11 days 5 h, Bouin fixed, on millimeter scale.
KT 949. 13:1

FIG. 151. Embryo of 11 days 5 h, Formol fixed, 5.3 mm length.
Explanation in drawing Fig. 152.
KT 950. 12.5:1

FIG. 152. Explanation of Fig. 151.
M = mesencephalon, S (*broken line*) = plane of section Fig. 153, *Tel* = hemisphere, $G 5$ = trigeminal ganglion, $G7$–8 = ganglia of 7th and 8th cranial nerves, O = otic vesicle, Aa = forelimb bud, Hl = hindlimb bud, 1 = mandibular process, 2 = hyoid arch.

FIG. 153. Eye anlage, frontal section, 11 days.
L = lens vesicle, in the process of closure; $A.c.$ = arteria carotis interna; Hy = enlarged vessel of hyaloid plexus; Ri = olfactory pit.
KT 605. 100:1

FIG. 154. Otic vesicle with endolymphatic duct (De).
Section parallel to S in drawing Fig. 152, same embryo of 11 days; Rh = wall of rhombencephalon; $V.c.a..$ = vena cardinalis anterior.
KT 605. 100:1

FIG. 155. Thyroid primordium, sagittal section, 11 days 5 h.
Th = ductus thyreoglossus (closed here).
KT 949/6. 560:1

FIG. 156. Placenta with 11 days 5 h.
Section of whole uterine wall. Embryo in situ. A = amnion, Au = arteria umbilicalis, D = yolk sac, visceral layer.
KT 951/3. 18:1

FIG. 157. Detail of Fig. 156.
La = labyrinth of placenta. eG = ectoplacental glycogen cells, Rz = trophoblastic giant cells. 100:1

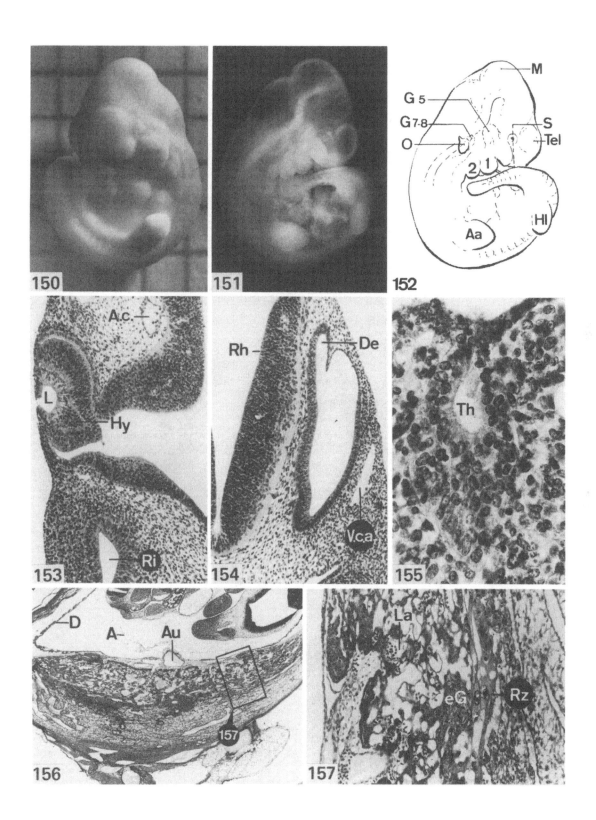

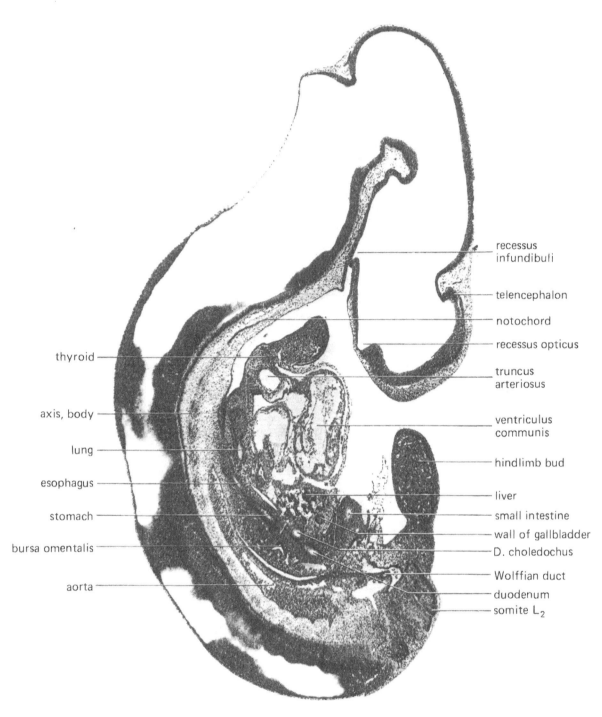

recessus
infundibuli

telencephalon

notochord

recessus opticus

truncus
arteriosus

ventriculus
communis

hindlimb bud

liver

small intestine

wall of gallbladder

D. choledochus

Wolffian duct

duodenum

somite L$_2$

thyroid

axis, body

lung

esophagus

stomach

bursa omentalis

aorta

FIG. 158. Sagittal section, 11 days 5 h, 5 mm length.
KT 949/6

Fig. 159. Section through upper thoracic region and anterior limb bud, 11 days 5 h. KT 951/3

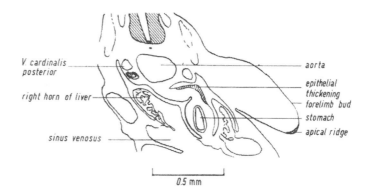

V. cardinalis posterior

right horn of liver

sinus venosus

aorta

epithelial thickening

forelimb bud

stomach

apical ridge

0.5 mm

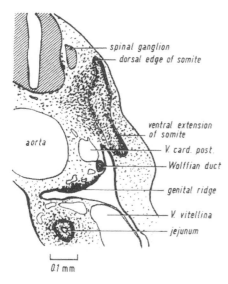

spinal ganglion

dorsal edge of somite

ventral extension of somite

V. card. post.

Wolffian duct

genital ridge

V. vitellina

jejunum

aorta

0.1 mm

Fig. 160. Cross section through lower thoracic region, 11 days 5 h. KT 951/3

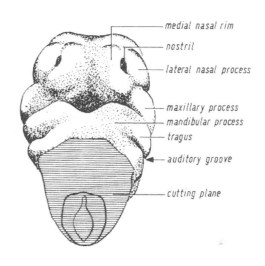

medial nasal rim

nostril

lateral nasal process

maxillary process

mandibular process

tragus

auditory groove

cutting plane

Fig. 162. Ventral view of the head, 11 days. Deep olfactory pit. Nasal folds fused posteriorly.

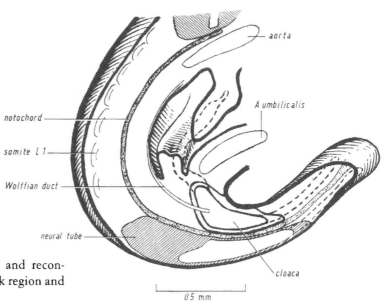

aorta

A. umbilicalis

notochord

somite L 1

Wolffian duct

neural tube

cloaca

0.5 mm

Fig. 161. Sagittal section and reconstruction of posterior trunk region and tail, 11 days. KT 605/2

Stage 19   Lens Vesicle Completely Separated from Surface

Horizon XVI
homo = 37 days
9–11 mm

11 1/2 Days, over 45 Somites, 6–7 mm

External Form

A footplate ("handplate") has formed in the anterior limb bud, indicated by a definite constriction (*arrow* in Fig. 163). The posterior limb buds are not yet divided into leg and foot. In the human, both hand- and footplates are delimited in horizon XVI (Streeter). Their development is dissimilar to that in the mouse, and they are less useful to use as landmarks to indicate developmental stage.

The six low tubercules, which will form the pinna, can be discerned.

The nostrils are narrowed to small slits, and the nasolacrimal grooves are clearly visible.

The posterior somites are still sharply defined, and the tail is considerably longer than in the preceding stage.

Length. Most are 6–7 mm long. A few specimens of this age group may be somewhat smaller (KT 611).

Sagittal section (Fig. 171): Compared with the preceding stage, there is little change in the brain. The opening of Rathke's pouch is constricted. The thyroid primordium is growing deeper and is losing its lumen. The mesenchyme of the anterior primitive intervertebral discs is condensing. In the lumbar region and posterior to it, there is a gradual transition from loose mesenchyme to condensation of the posterior sclerotomic halves of the somites. The atlas is visible in Fig. 175.

Circulatory System

Within the *arterial system*, the aortic arch complex has become more mature (Fig. 172). The most anterior arch has disappeared, and the second is reduced. The third and sixth are well developed. All of them connect dorsally with the dorsal aorta. The vertebral artery is now forming parallel to the dorsal aorta. The primitive arteria cerebri anterior (olfactory artery) has enlarged considerably along with the further development of the nose.

In the *venous system*, the asymmetry of the umbilical veins is striking. The sinus venosus receives the cardinal veins, the right umbilical vein and the hepato-cardiac channel (primitive inferior vena cava) (Fig. 173). The sinus venosus conducts the blood through a small sinuatrial opening into the atrium.

The *atrium* is nearly completely partitioned off by the septum primum. The original broad communication is constricted to the foramen I, while the foramen II is forming above (Fig. 174).

The *ventricle* is still unpaired (ventriculus communis). It is delimited from the atrium by the atrio-ventricular cushions (Fig. 175). This figure illustrates how the arterial outlet is incompletely subdivided by the developing bulbar ridges. It also shows how the pulmonary artery branches off as a thin vessel from the sixth aortic arch. The opening of the sixth aortic arch into the large dorsal aorta is also visible in Fig. 175.

Intestinal Tract

In the region of the *foregut*, the elevation of the tongue is not yet apparent. Anterior to the foramen cecum, there is a small indentation (Fig. 176), which must not be confused with it. The thyroid primordium has invaded more deeply into the underlying mesenchyme (Figs. 171 and 176), and the primary (stem) bronchi are developing secondary branches (lobar bronchi). Lung lobation is determined genetically [61].

The pharyngeal pouches are now beginning to become specialized structures such as the thymus and parathyroid. They are not yet completely separated from the pharyngeal epithelium.

The *stomach* is much enlarged. It is separated from the outgrowing pancreas by the lesser sac (bursa omentalis). The *liver* is composed of broad hepatic cords, which are separated by large sinusoids containing nucleated erythrocytes. Hematopoietic foci are found intermingled with the hepatic cords.

The *cecum* is recognizable by a slight distension of the colon. It marks a clear distinction between colon and small intestine. Within the cloaca the uro-rectal septum is developing (Figs. 176 and 177). The cloacal membrane has not yet ruptured. Posteriorly, the hindgut is continued by the tail gut, which terminates in the blastema of the tail tip. The tail gut is very narrow, except for a slight terminal distension, and it has some pycnotic cells. The ventral ectodermal ridge [186] is confined to the region near the tail tip.

Urogenital System

The urogenital system is developing rapidly. The genital ridge, still in an indifferent state, contains numerous gonocytes (Fig. 168), which have now completed their migration [103]. The Wolffian ducts terminate blindly at the cloaca. The ureteric buds are considerably distended. They are surrounded by condensed metanephrogenic tissue [100] (Figs. 167 and 177). The *mesonephros* is more mature than in the preceding stage. Several glomerulusanlagen may now be recognized, and the mesonephric tubules are more distinct (Fig. 178).

Central Nervous System

Eye. The most conspicuous feature of this age group is the complete closure of the lens vesicle and its detachment from the ectoderm (Fig. 166).

The pigment layer of the optic cup contains numerous cells with pigment granules.

Ear. The endolymphatic duct is longer, and the utricle and saccule are becoming discernible.

Olfactory organ. The nose pit is separated from the oral cavity by the bucco-nasal membrane (Fig. 179). The epithelial wall of Hochstetter is invaded and perforated by mesenchyme (Fig. 169). In the medial wall, the invaginated organ of Jacobson is clearly visible.

The *ganglia* of the cranial nerves and the spinal ganglia are well developed and the anlage of the *sympathetic trunk* is discernible (Fig. 175).

The cellular degeneration, which began at 10 1/2 days in the anterior part of the roof of the 3rd ventricle, has progressed further.

Extraembryonic membranes. In the yolk sac, numerous well-vascularized superficial folds have formed.

Material	Age	
KT 1004–6	11 days 10 h	6 embryos, 6.1–6.5 mm (unfixed)
		1 resorption
KT 630–31	12 days	7 embryos, 6–7 mm (copulation age advanced)
KT 611–12	11 days 21 h	4 embryos, 5–5.5 mm
		2 embryos, 2–2.5 mm (hypoplastic)

FIG. 163. Embryo, right side, on millimeter scale, 11 1/2 days (nt 114).
Arrow indicates indentation delimiting the forefoot-plate. 9:1

FIG. 164. Embryo, left side, explanation in drawing Fig. 165 (nt 114). 9:1

FIG. 165. Explanation of Fig. 164.
Tel = cerebral hemisphere, M = mesencephalon, Ns = nostrils, Rh = rhombencephalon, Tr = nasolacrimal groove, *1, 2* = branchial bars, *V.c.a.* = vena cardinalis anterior, He = heart (ventricle), So = somite (1st lumbar), Aa = forelimb bud, Hl = hindlimb bud, L_3 = spinal ganglion (3rd lumbar), L = lens vesicle (just closed).

FIG. 166. Eye, frontal section.
A.c. = arteria cerebri anterior, Pi = pigment epithelium, R = retinal layer, Hy = hyaloid plexus, L = lens vesicle (just closed).
KT 630a/6. 130:1

FIG. 167. Caudal end of Wolffian duct, with ureteric bud.
Coe = coelom, Ur = ureteric bud, W = Wolffian duct, Me = metanephrogenic tissue.
KT 630b/3. 130:1

FIG. 168. Sagittal section through germinal ridge.
Coe = coelom, Ge = gonocyte.
KT 630b/6. 700:1

FIG. 169. Cross section through forebrain and olfactory apparatus.
A = anterior section, nostril; B = intermediate section: dissolution of epithelial wall; *Tel* = telencephalon; Sc = tail, cross sectioned; J = vomeronasal organ (Jacobson).
KT 630a/7. 40:1

FIG. 170. Cross section through forebrain and olfactory apparatus.
C = posterior section with bucconasal membrane, Tr = nasolacrimal groove, *C.s.* = corpus striatum, Sc = tail.
KT 630a/7. 40:1

80

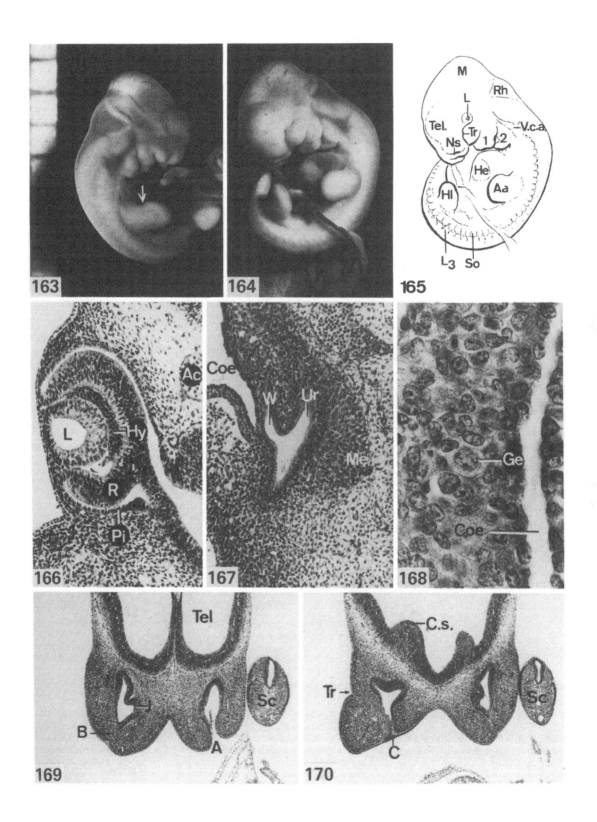

81

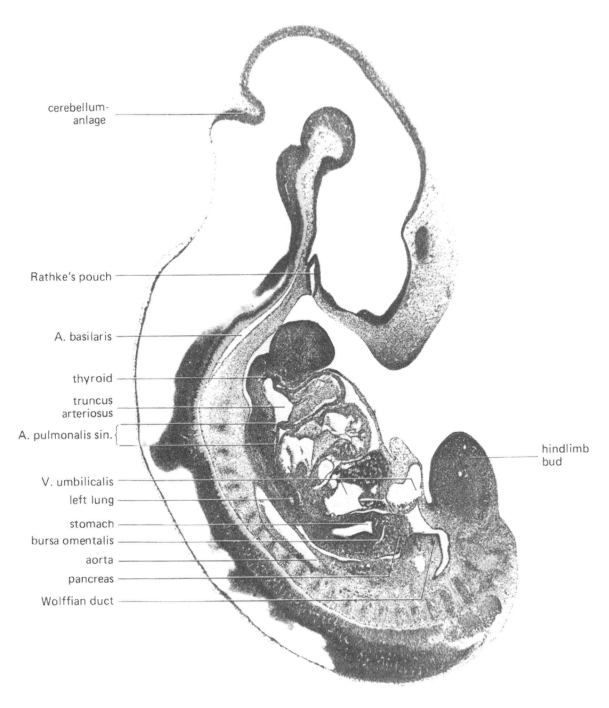

cerebellum-
anlage

Rathke's pouch

A. basilaris

thyroid

truncus
arteriosus

A. pulmonalis sin. {

V. umbilicalis

left lung

stomach

bursa omentalis

aorta

pancreas

Wolffian duct

hindlimb
bud

FIG. 171. Sagittal section, 11 days 10 h, 6.3 mm length.
KT 1005

82

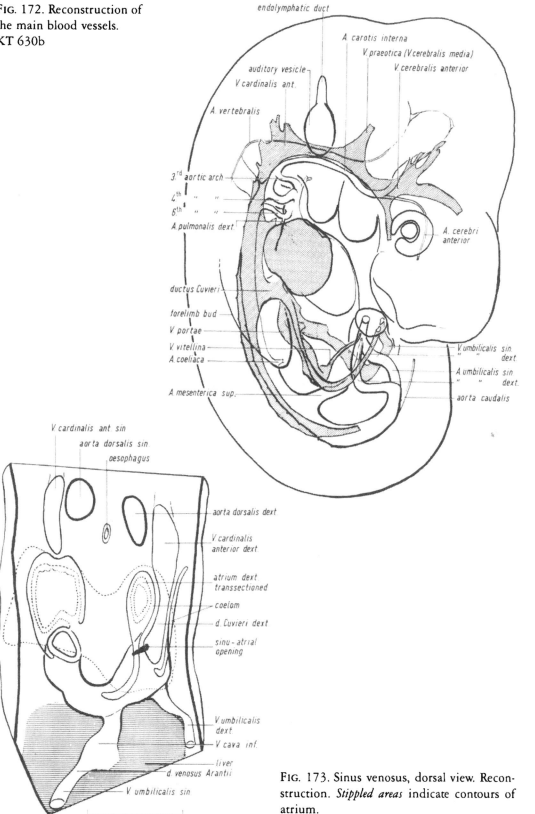

FIG. 172. Reconstruction of
the main blood vessels.
KT 630b

endolymphatic duct

A carotis interna
V. praeotica (V cerebralis media)
V. cerebralis anterior

auditory vesicle
V. cardinalis ant.

A. vertebralis

3.rd aortic arch
4.th " "
6.th " "
A. pulmonalis dext.

A. cerebri
anterior

ductus Cuvieri

forelimb bud
V. portae
V. vitellina
A. coeliaca

A. mesenterica sup.

V. umbilicalis sin.
" " dext.
A. umbilicalis sin.
" " dext.
aorta caudalis

V. cardinalis ant. sin
aorta dorsalis sin
oesophagus

aorta dorsalis dext

V. cardinalis
anterior dext.

atrium dext
transsectioned
coelom
d. Cuvieri dext

sinu-atrial
opening

V. umbilicalis
dext.
V. cava inf.

liver
d. venosus Arantii
V. umbilicalis sin

0.5 m m

FIG. 173. Sinus venosus, dorsal view. Reconstruction. *Stippled areas* indicate contours of
atrium.
KT 630c/4

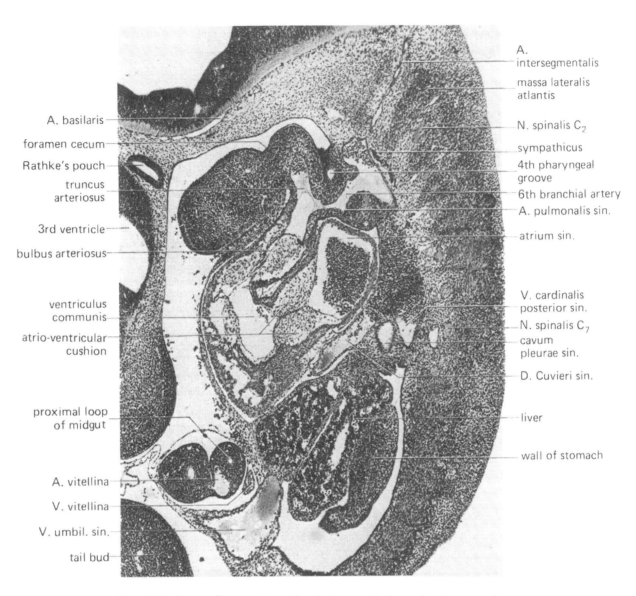

A. basilaris

foramen cecum

Rathke's pouch

truncus
arteriosus

3rd ventricle

bulbus arteriosus

ventriculus
communis

atrio-ventricular
cushion

proximal loop
of midgut

A. vitellina

V. vitellina

V. umbil. sin.

tail bud

A.
intersegmentalis

massa lateralis
atlantis

N. spinalis C_2

sympathicus

4th pharyngeal
groove

6th branchial artery

A. pulmonalis sin.

atrium sin.

V. cardinalis
posterior sin.

N. spinalis C_7

cavum
pleurae sin.

D. Cuvieri sin.

liver

wall of stomach

Fig. 175. Paramedian section. Nominal age 12 days, developmentally
11 1/2 days.
KT 630b

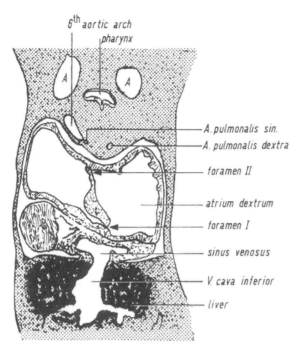

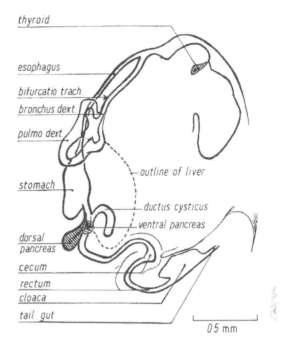

FIG. 174. Septation of atrium, frontal section, dorsal view.
A = aorta dorsalis (paired).
KT 630c/4

FIG. 176. Intestinal tract, reconstruction.
KT 630b, 6 mm, developmental age 11 1/2 days

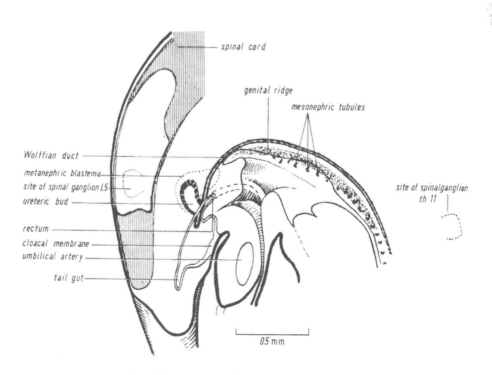

FIG. 177. Urogenital apparatus, left half, reconstructed.
KT 630b

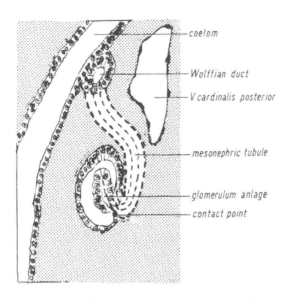

FIG. 178. Differentiation of mesonephros. Cross section.
KT 630a, developmental age 11 1/2 days

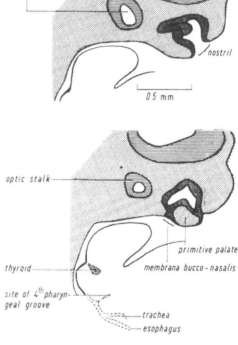

FIG. 179. Development of olfactory apparatus.
Lateral section (*above*) and medial section (*below*), in sagittal direction.
KT 630b, developmental age 11 1/2 days

FIG. 180. Sagittal section through fore- and midbrain.
KT 1005/1, 11 1/2 days. 40:1

FIG. 181. Detail of Fig. 180. Disintegrating cells in the anterior roof of the diencephalon. 560:1

Stage 20   Earliest Signs of Fingers
12 Days, 7–9 mm

External Form

The most conspicuous changes take place in the extremities. The "handplate" is no longer roundish. Even in younger members of this group there is a slightly angular contour (Fig. 182). The developing angles correspond to the finger rays [184]. The posterior footplate is now demarcated from the lower part of the leg. The somites are clearly visible from the tail to the mid-trunk region. The spinal ganglia may be seen through the skin in transparent specimens.

Length. 7–9 mm, measured in a direct crown-rump line.

Circulatory System

Arteries. The second aortic arch has disappeared. The third, fourth, and sixth are of variable caliber, but symmetric (Fig. 191).

Heart. The truncus arteriosus is being partitioned. The septum membranaceum is still incomplete.

The septation of the atrium (Fig. 192) began in the preceding period. This important event is illustrated in Figs. 193–196. These sections were taken from embryo KT 630. Its nominal age is 12 days, but its developmental age is 11 1/2 days.

Intestinal Tract

Profound transformations in the intestinal tract are occurring.

In the *pharyngeal region*, the anlage of the *tongue* is delimited from the lower jaw by a furrow (Fig. 190).

The anlagen of the *teeth* appear as slight epithelial thickenings. A continuous dental lamina is not apparent anteriorly [76].

Lateral to the mid-sagittal plane, the furrow in front of the tongue gives rise to the out-budding ductus submaxillaris.

The *thyroid primordium* is closely attached to the arcus aortae. It is displaced very deep and its connection with the slight indentation of the foramen caecum is becoming indistinct (Fig. 197, *dashed line*). The cells of the thyroid are strongly eosinophilic. Sometimes, they seem to form rosettes. True formation of follicles, however, does not occur until a much later phase [147]. The third and fourth *pharyngeal pouches* are now budding out. The 3rd produces the thymus and parathyroid anlage [146]. They still connect with the pharyngeal epithelium, but the uniting epithelial bridges contain many decaying cells.

The fourth pouch yields the so-called ultimo-branchial body [146].

The *lung buds* (Figs. 188 and 189) have not only secondary (lobar), but tertiary (segmental) bronchi. The pleural cavity is in broad communication with the peritoneal cavity (Fig. 198, ductus pleuro-peritonealis).

The stomach is greatly distended, and there are regional differences in the epithelium (Fig. 188). Both rudiments of the pancreas are in contact with each other.

Within the *liver*, there are megakaryocytes, and as previously mentioned, blood is being formed.

Urogenital Tract

The *mesonephros* contains distinct tubules, but no well-formed glomeruli. Evidently mesonephric glomeruli remain primitive in mice, and perhaps they never function.

The *metanephros* has only two polar tubes (pelvic poles) in younger specimens (KT 643/2), but many secondary buds in older (KT 634/8) specimens of this group [102].

The *ureter* is relatively narrow and opens into the Wolffian duct, which still ends blindly within the epithelium of the urogenital sinus.

The uro-rectal septum has not yet reached the cloacal membrane (Fig. 198).

FIG. 182. Embryo, from the right. Albino of a control series, fixed, on millimeter scale.
Tr = nasolacrimal groove.
10:1

FIG. 183. Embryo from the left, life photograph.
KT 942, 11 days 23 h. 9:1

FIG. 184. Explanation of Fig. 183.
0 = otic vesicle, *NS* = nostril, *F* = choroid fissure, *I.* = first branchial pouch, *Hl* = hindlimb bud,
Tr = nasolacrimal groove.

FIG. 185. Eye, frontal section.
Pi = pigment epithelium, *Lf* = lens fibers.
KT 943/11, 12 days. 130:1

FIG. 186. Primordium of vertebral column, thoracic region. Frontal section.
N = spinal nerve, *Iv* = intersegmental vessels, *If* = intrasegmental fissure (sclerotomic fissure),
a = cranial sclerotomic half, *b* = caudal sclerotomic half, *CH* = notochord.
KT 941/3, 12 days, 8 mm length. 100:1

FIG. 187. Sagittal section through cervical ganglia.
N XII = nervus hypoglossus, *Gc2* = ganglion cervicale 2, *At* = atlas, *A.v.* = arteria vertebralis.
35:1

FIG. 188. Sagittal section through lower thoracic and abdominal region.
Oe = esophagus, *St* = stomach, *Li* = liver, *Pa* = pancreas, *K* = kidney, *Sy* = sympathetic trunk,
Ths = caput costae 5, *V* = vena cardinalis posterior sinistra.
KT 943/8, 12 days. 40:1

FIG. 189. Detail of Fig. 188.
Lu = left lung, *Sp* = nervus splanchnicus, *NN* = suprarenal gland. 100:1

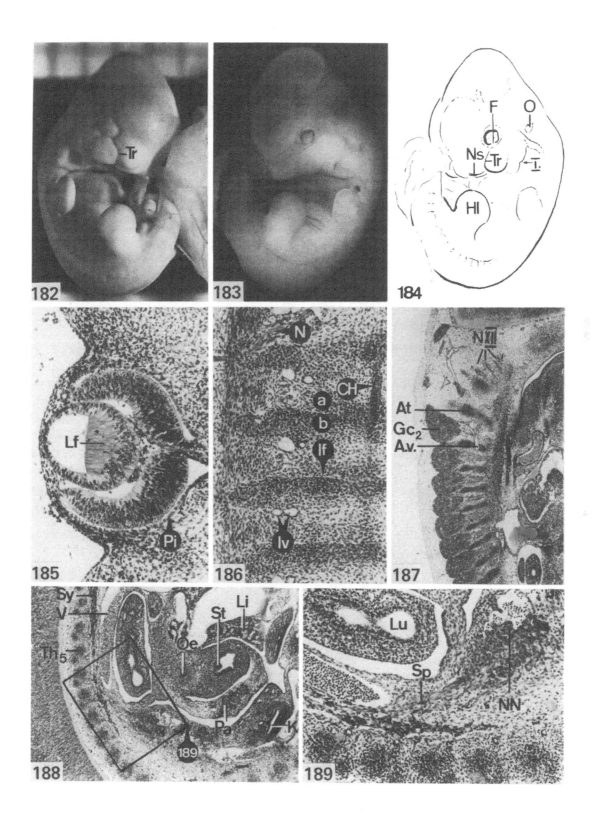

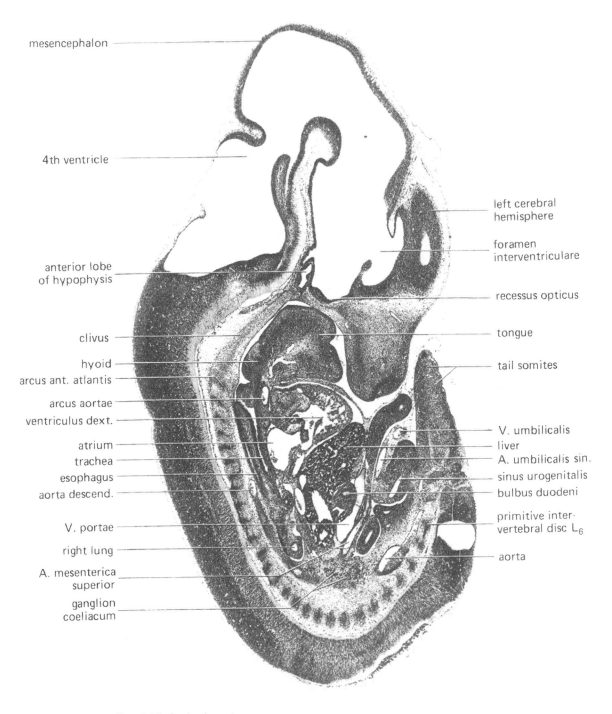

mesencephalon

4th ventricle

left cerebral
hemisphere

foramen
interventriculare

anterior lobe
of hypophysis

recessus opticus

clivus

tongue

hyoid

tail somites

arcus ant. atlantis

arcus aortae

ventriculus dext.

V. umbilicalis

atrium

liver

trachea

A. umbilicalis sin.

esophagus

sinus urogenitalis

aorta descend.

bulbus duodeni

V. portae

primitive inter-
vertebral disc L$_6$

right lung

aorta

A. mesenterica
superior

ganglion
coeliacum

FIG. 190. Sagittal section.
KT 943/8, 12 days, 8 mm length

90

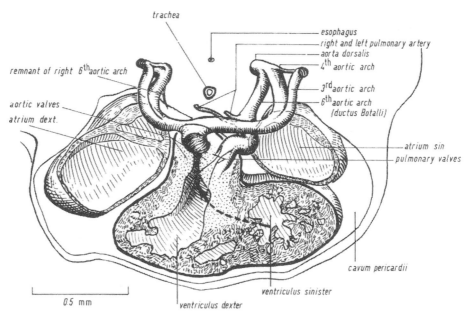

FIG. 191. Frontal section and reconstruction of the arterial trunk.
Arrow indicates the aortal pathway. Septum membranaceum still incomplete. Beginning formation of semilunar valves.
KT 943/11, 12 days

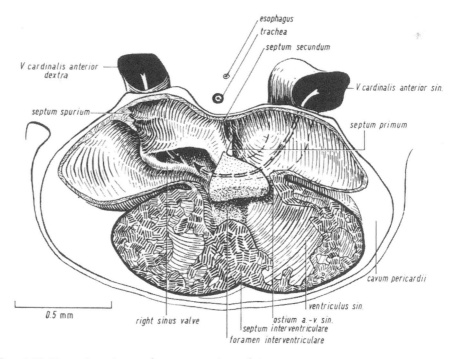

FIG. 192. Frontal section and reconstruction of the atrium.
Arrows indicate the blood flow of the sinus venosus. *Clear area* indicates upper atrioventricular cushion; *stippled area* indicates lower cushion.
KT 943/11, 12 days

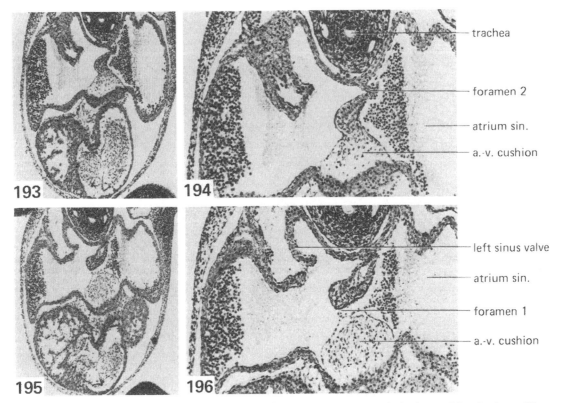

FIG. 193–196. Low and medium magnification of cross sections through the heart. Nominal age 12 days. Formation of foramen primum and secundum.
KT 630, 55:1 and 100:1

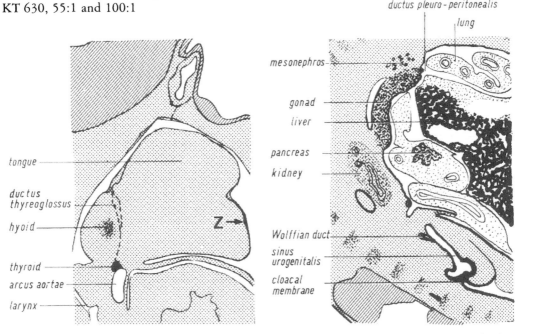

FIG. 197. Sagittal section of oral and pharyngeal region with thyroid primordium.

The thyreo-glossal duct (*broken line*) is interrupted; Z indicates thickening of the mandibular epithelium. Lip furrow and lower incisivus will develop from here.

FIG. 198. Urogenital apparatus, sagittal section.
KT 943/8, 12 days, 8 mm length

FIG. 199. Reconstruction of the labyrinth, sagittal section. The major part of the lateral and upper semicircular ducts are cut away.

KT 943/7, 12 days, 8 mm length

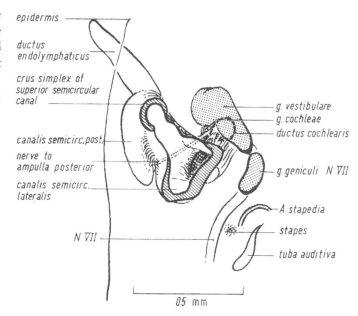

The *gonads* are still in the indifferent state (Fig. 198). Sexual differentiation is usually apparent histologically at 12 1/2 days and sometimes at 12 days [118].

The *suprarenal* is distinct and is composed of cellular cords representing the cortex [137] (Fig. 189).

Central Nervous System

In this phase, the pineal gland appears as a discrete evagination in the most posterior part of the diencephalic roof (not visible in the section shown in Fig. 190). In the anterior part of the roof, near the interventricular foramen, there are still numerous pycnoses [166].

Eye. The posterior wall of the lens vesicle is markedly thickened as a result of differentiation of lens fibers (Fig. 185).

Otocyst. The subdivisions of the labyrinth are easily recognized. The semicircular canals, however, are still flat pouches, which are not yet tubular. The cochlear duct is short (Fig. 199, *dashed line*). The vestibular ganglion has larger cells than the cochlear ganglion (most of which is hidden in Fig. 199).

The auditory capsules still consists of mesenchyme, which will soon chondrify.

Material	Age	
KT 620–21	11 days 22 h	6 embryos: 8, 8, 8.5, 8.5, 8.8 mm
KT 941–43	11 days 23 h	5 embryos: 7.6–8.3 mm
KT 622–23	12 days	7 embryos: 7, 7.5, 8.2, 8.6, 9, 9, 9.1 mm
KT 628	12 days 3 h	5 embryos: 6–8 mm
KT 629	12 days 3 h	6 embryos: approximately 8 mm
KT 636	12 days 2 h	7 embryos: 7.5–8.7 mm

Stage 21 Anterior Footplate Indented; Marked Pinna

13 Days, 9–11 mm

Horizon XVIII–XIX
homo = 44–48 days
14–20 mm

Externally. The rapid development of the *pinna* is striking, and it now forms a crest at right angles to the head. Five rows of whiskers are present. The 4 upper rows of whiskers are shown in Fig. 202, as well as a prominent hair follicle above the eye and another in front of the ear. The indentation of the *handplate* is characteristic of this period. It is shallow in younger embryos of this stage (Fig. 200) and very distinct in older ones (Fig. 201). The footplate is just becoming indented.

Somites are clearly visible only in the distal part of the tail. Usually the tail is curved to the left (as in Fig. 202) rather than to the right.

Length. The length varies from 9–11 mm in unfixed embryos.

Sagittal section (Fig. 208). In the brain, the choroid plexus projects into the lateral and the 4th ventricle, forming finger-like evaginations. The tongue projects from the floor of the mouth {76}.

Locomotive System

The extremities now differentiate rapidly [184]. As shown in Fig. 209, the skeleton of the forelimb already contains cartilage, while the "hand" still remains mesenchymous. The cranial vertebrae are chondrified, but not the more posterior ones.

Circulatory System

The aortic and pulmonary trunks are completely separated as shown in Fig. 208. The membranous part of the interventricular septum is not yet closed. Within the coronary sulcus, fine coronary vessels are visible. There is probably not yet a continuous circulation. All valves of the heart are now present in primitive form.

The inferior caval vein is represented proximally by a large hepato-cardiac channel. The venous system is essentially the same, as that shown in the reconstruction (Fig. 224) made for the next developmental phase (14 days).

Intestinal Tract

The *oral cavity* is in broad communication with the nasal cavity. The palatine processes consist of mesenchyme and are in a vertical position. The dental lamina of the future molars is clearly visible [73] (Fig. 210).

In sagittal sections (Fig. 208) the *epiglottis* is delimited by a discrete cleft from the rest of the larynx, which projects plug-like into the pharynx.

The *lungs* are clearly subdivided into lobes [61], and the segmental bronchi are continuing to branch.

The *thymus* has completely lost its connection with the pharynx. Numerous blood vessels are penetrating the thymus primordium, but the closely neighboring and considerably smaller *thyroid* is still a solid complex [147].

Within the abdomen, the *liver* is well developed and contains scattered blood-forming foci. The stomach does not yet have differentiated glands. In some places the epithelium is higher than in others, and there are some small lumina (Fig. 208). The spleen appears in cross sections as a triangular structure (Fig. 206).

The pancreas produces numerous sprouts, which considerably swell the dorsal mesentery (Fig. 208).

Urogenital Tract

The urogenital tract is characterized by the rapid development of the *kidney* and by *sexual differentiation.*

The mesonephros contains many regressing mesonephric tubules (Fig. 204). The slender ureter is continuous with the distended pelvis, which has well-marked primary calyces with caps of metanephric tissue (Fig. 206). The metanephric caps [100], in some places, form small vesicles, which are more intensely eosinophilic than the ureteric bud. The vesicles are sometimes transformed into S-shaped tubules, the free ends of which have differentiating glomeruli. The *Wolffian duct* is more developed in the male, the *Müllerian duct* more in the female. The cloaca is completely subdivided. The ureter has contact both with the Wolffian duct and with the urogenital sinus. It still ends blindly, slightly cranial to the lower end of the mesonephric duct.

The sex of the gonads can now be diagnosed. In the male, the future seminiferous tubules appear as solid, regularly arranged strands [118]. They are composed of small supporting and nourishing cells, and of large primordial germ cells (Fig. 207). The first suggestion of sexual differentiation appeared at 12 1/2 days. Male primordial germ cells were located centrally, and female germ cells were located peripherally. Some of the large female gonocytes (Fig. 205) are dividing.

Central Nervous System

There are pronounced changes in the diencephalic roof (Fig. 211). There are no longer pycnotic cells in the anterior portion of the roof [166]. The choroid plexus is fully developed. The *pineal gland* was recognizable at 12 days as a small evagination, and it is now very distinct. The posterior commissure is also well formed [160].

The *hypophysis* is developing very rapidly (Figs. 212–214).

The structure of the *eye* is very characteristic for this group: the lens vesicle has lost its lumen, and is a solid sphere. The vitreous body is exceedingly small. In the retina, the layer of nerve fibers forms a wide border with peripherally tapering ends. The nuclear layers of the retina are still predominantly indistinguishable from each other. However, the clear nuclei of the future ganglionic cells are discernible in some places. The ganglion cell layer is the first one to be delimited from the other layers.

Material	Age	
KT 615–16	12 days 23 h	7 embryos, 10–11 mm
KT 633–34	13 days 3 h	6 embryos, 10–10.8 mm
KT 1014–16	13 days 2 h	8 embryos + 1 resorption, about 10 mm
KT 901	12 days 20 h	7 embryos, 9.6–10.0 mm (after fixation)

FIG. 200. Embryo from the right. Younger stage of 12 days 6 h. Formalin fixed.
Ey = eye, *Tel* = cerebral hemisphere.
KT 952, 8.7 mm length. 8:1

FIG. 201. Embryo from the left, 13 days, 10 mm length, life photograph.
Si = sinus sigmoideus.
KT 634. 7:1

FIG. 202. Frontal view. Albino of control series. Bouin fixed, 13 days, 10 mm length.
O = pinna, *So* = tail somites, *N* = nostril, *H* = rudiments of hair follicles (whiskers). 10:1

FIG. 203. Eye, cross section, 13 days.
OL = upper lid, *L* = lens, *St* = optic stalk, *P* = pigment layer. 70:1

FIG. 204. Ovary and vicinity. Cross section, 13 days.
NN = suprarenal gland, *U* = mesonephric tubules, *M* = Müllerian duct, *Ma* = stomach.
KT 901/5. 100:1

FIG. 205. Detail of Fig. 204.
Oz = oocytes in meiotic prophase. 550:1

FIG. 206. Testis and vicinity, 13 days.
NN = suprarenal gland, *Ur* = ureter in kidney rudiment, *W* = Wolffian duct, *M* = Müllerian duct, *B* = omental bursa, bordering the triangular anlage of the spleen (*right*) and the stomach (*below*).
KT 901/2

FIG. 207. Detail of Fig. 206, testis.
Sp = Gonocytes. 550:1

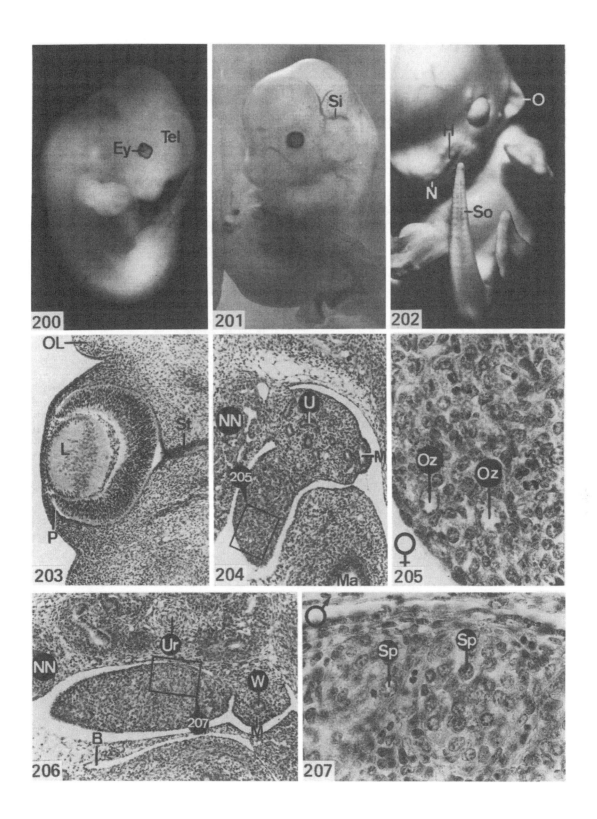

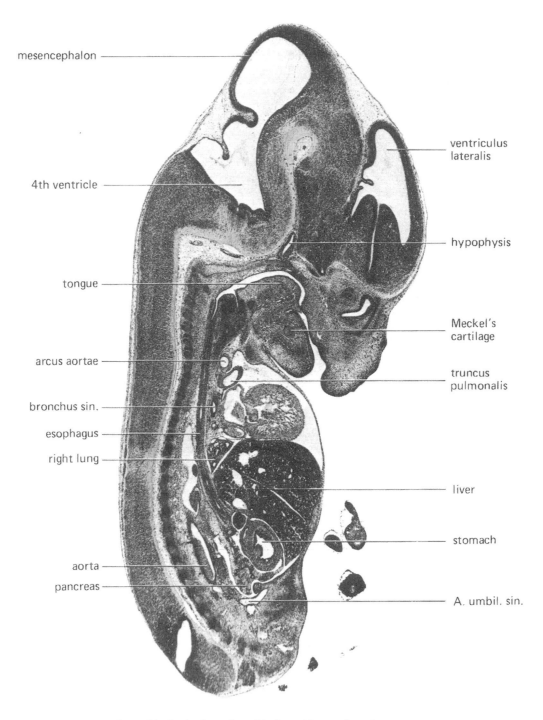

mesencephalon

ventriculus
lateralis

4th ventricle

hypophysis

tongue

Meckel's
cartilage

arcus aortae

truncus
pulmonalis

bronchus sin.

esophagus

right lung

liver

stomach

aorta

pancreas

A. umbil. sin.

FIG. 208. Sagittal section, 13 days, 10 mm length.
KT 901/2

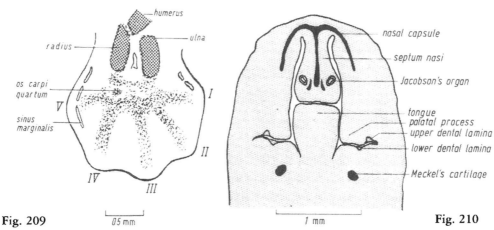

Fig. 209   Fig. 210

Fig. 209. ▲
Right forefoot plate, 13 days.
Dark stippled area indicates precartilage (of "arm" skeleton); *light stippled area* indicates mesenchymal condensations.
KT 1014

Fig. 210. Cross section through oral and nasal cavities. Plane of section nearly horizontal, therefore the conchae are not visible.
Black area indicates cartilage and precartilage.
KT 901, 12 days 2 h

Fig. 211. ———————————————▶
Sagittal section through roof of diencephalon.
E = epiphysis, *Co* = commissura posterior, *For i.v.* = foramen interventriculare.
KT 633/b, 13 days

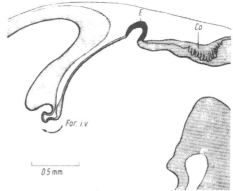

Fig. 211

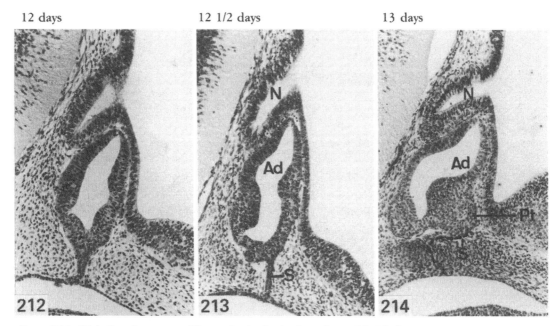

12 days   12 1/2 days   13 days

212   213   214

Figs. 212–214. Development of hypophysis. Sagittal sections, 12–13 days.
N = neurohypophysis, *Ad* = adenohypophysis, *P.t.* = pars tuberalis, *S* = connecting stalk (with pharyngeal roof).

Stage 22   Fingers Separate Distally
14 Days, 11–12 mm

Externally. With magnification, one can easily see that the individual *fingers* are separated in the forefoot plate. In contrast, in the hindfoot plate there are deep indentations between the developing toes, but they are not yet separated (Figs. 215–217). Numerous young *hair follicles* may be recognized in the skin, except for the head region. The *somites* are discernible only in the distal part of the tail. The growing pinna is turned forward and covers about one-half of the external auditory meatus. The umbilical hernia is very conspicuous at this stage (Fig. 216 and 217).

Length. The length varies from 10.4 to 12 mm.

Circulatory System

Arteries. Both *umbilical arteries* are united at the umbilical ring to form a single vessel, which passes through the umbilical cord (not visible in Fig. 224).

The arterial system of the *head* is being transformed. In Fig. 224, the *arteria stapedia* is recognizable. It is a branch of the second aortic arch. The stump of the right pulmonary artery is visible below the ductus arteriosus Botalli. The right fourth aortic arch has lost its communication with the dorsal aorta, and flows directly into the artery of the right forelimb (arteria subclavia dextra). On the whole, the definitive pattern of the prenatal circulatory system is established, and the definitive shape of the heart as well. The ventricular septum is now closed.

Veins. The *cardinal veins* are markedly asymmetrical. The posterior cardinal vein as shown in Fig. 224 is the original *left* posterior cardinal vein, while the right has regressed (in the reconstruction of a 12-day stage—Fig. 172—both are present). The anterior cardinals are both present and will persist in the adult mouse.

Intestinal Tract

The palatal processes are elevating and begin to separate the oral and nasal cavities (Figs. 225 and 226). They are not yet fused, so that the cavities are still continuous. Occasionally, the fusion of the palatal processes may be delayed and the tongue appears to be squeezed between them (Fig. 223). The posterior part of the open communication in Fig. 225 always remains open. With progressive growth, this communication will be displaced posteriorly and form a long duct (ductus naso-pharyngeus).

The bud of the first *molar* [73] is visible (Fig. 226). The second and third will appear later. In sagittal section (Fig. 223), the anlagen of the lower and upper incisors [76] may be recognized (not labeled). They are located above and beneath the tip of the tongue.

Meckel's and Reichert's cartilage are more advanced in development than the precartilaginous skeleton of the *larynx*. The tracheal rings are still mesenchymal condensations.

The *thymus* and *thyroid* are easily recognizable (Fig. 223). The thymus has lost its connection with the third pharyngeal pouch, and is situated above the pericardium. The parathyroids are joining the thyroid [146].

The bronchi are considerably distended and have numerous ramifications (Fig. 223).

The gut projects into the wide umbilical hernial sac. The mucosal lining of the gut consists of relatively tall columnar cells. The configuration of the intestinal tract is represented in Fig. 227.

Urogenital System

The *ureter* now opens into the urogenital sinus separately from the opening of the Wolffian duct. The sinus itself has been separated from the rectum in an earlier phase of development. The topography of the embryonic urogenital system is represented in Fig. 228, and microscopic details are shown in Fig. 223.

Sexual differentiation is very apparent: the seminiferous tubules are solid strands of cells, which are nearly symmetrically arranged [118] (Fig. 221). The ovary, on the other hand, does not form cords [122]. In the female, the Müllerian duct is now more highly developed than the Wolffian duct (Fig. 219).

Central Nervous System

In the *telencephalon* cells migrate from the mantle zone and form a *superficial cortical layer* (primary cortex). It is separated from the broad mantle zone by a thin marginal zone, with few nuclei (Fig. 223). The choroid plexus of the lateral ventricle projects far into the lumen. All cranial nerves are now distinctly visible, and the ganglia are relatively large (Fig. 229).

Eye. The cavity of the vitreous body has increased considerably in size. The ganglionic layer of the retina (not the bipolar layer) appears as a zone of clear nuclei. It is distinguishable from the two darker inner zones, which are not yet separated from each other. The separation occurs much later, after birth.

The eyelids are prominent.

Ear. The ductus cochlearis has elongated and it curves to form a full circle. It is bordered by a thin cartilaginous capsule. The presumptive sensory epithelium may be recognized by its height.

Hypophysis (Fig. 230–232). The connecting strand of epithelial cells (marked *S* in Fig. 214) has disappeared. The pars tuberalis continues to elongate. Ventral to the hypophysis is the cartilaginous base of the skull.

Placenta (Figs. 233–234). The labyrinth reached the peak of its development at 12 days.

The development of the so-called "yolk sac diverticles" is a conspicuous characteristic of this stage. They arise as clefts within the trophoblastic labyrinth and may perforate it [33] (Fig. 234). The visceral (proximal) layer of the yolk sac has many branching folds.

Material	Age	
KT 618	13 days 21 h	4 embryos, 11–11.5 mm
KT 642–44	14 days	7 embryos, 11.5–12 mm (1 of them exencephalic)
KT 659–660	14 days	5 embryos, 10.5–12 mm
KT 1017–22	14 days 2 h	5 embryos, 10.6–11.9 mm
KT 1043–45	14 days 4 1/2 h	4 embryos, 10.4–11.3 mm

FIG. 215. Embryo from the left. Life photograph.
KT 642, 14 days, 12 mm length. 6:1

FIG. 216. Embryo from the left (albino of control series). Bouin fixed, 14 days, 11 mm length.
6.6:1

FIG. 217. Explanation of Fig. 216.
O = pinna; *H* = hair follicles; *Fi* = finger, separated; *Nb* = umbilical hernia; *So* = tail somites.

FIG. 218. Horizonal section through eye.
G = ganglion nervi optici, *K* = nuclear layers (dark), *P* = pigmented layer.
KT 643, 14 days. 55:1

FIG. 219. Ovary and vicinity, sagittal section.
W = Wolffian duct, *M* = Müllerian duct, *U* = mesonephric tubules, *Ma* = stomach, *DM* = Dorsal mesogastrium.
KT 643b, 14 days. 100:1

FIG. 220. Detail of Fig. 219.
Oz = oocyte, *Ep* = epithelium, *Er* = erythrocyte in capillary. 700:1

FIG. 221. Testis, tangential section. Seminiferous tubules, solid, nearly symmetrical arrangement.
Li = liver.
KT 643a, 14 days. 135:1

FIG. 222. Enlarged view of seminiferous tubule.
Sp = gonocyte, in prophase. 700:1

102

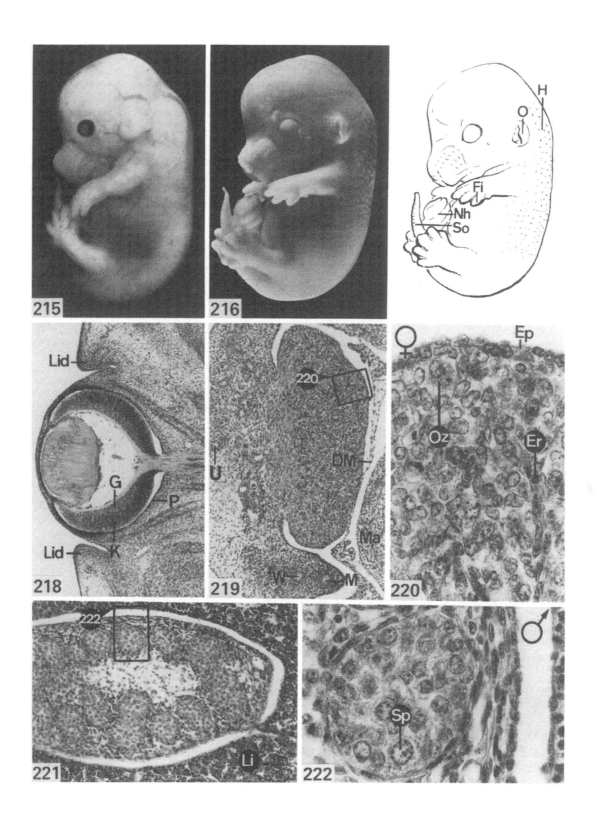

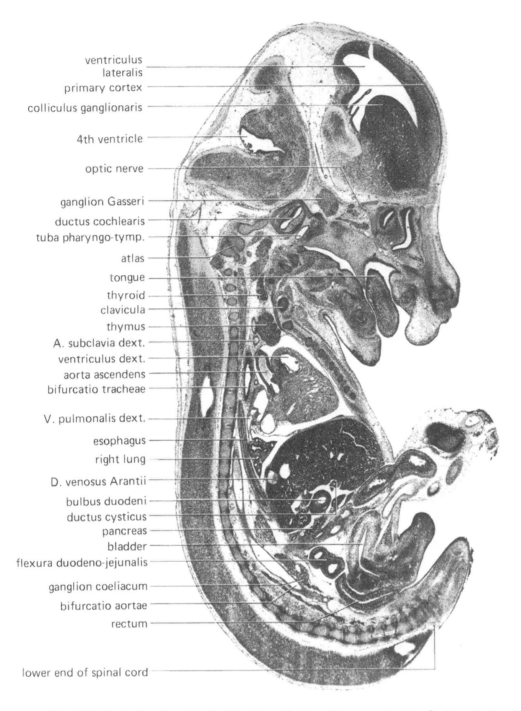

ventriculus
lateralis
primary cortex
colliculus ganglionaris

4th ventricle

optic nerve

ganglion Gasseri
ductus cochlearis
tuba pharyngo-tymp.

atlas
tongue
thyroid
clavicula
thymus
A. subclavia dext.
ventriculus dext.
aorta ascendens
bifurcatio tracheae

V. pulmonalis dext.

esophagus

right lung

D. venosus Arantii

bulbus duodeni
ductus cysticus
pancreas
bladder
flexura duodeno-jejunalis

ganglion coeliacum

bifurcatio aortae

rectum

lower end of spinal cord

FIG. 223. Sagittal section, female. The choroid plexus is now projecting far into the lateral ventricle. The wall of the hemisphere, which is cut here, shows peripherally a small primary *cortical layer*. The vertebral column has become chondrified. It contains relatively big notochordal segments. Some of them are visible in the thoracic region of the section (Fig. 223). At the base of the tail they are still small.

KT 643b, 14 days, 11.5 mm

104

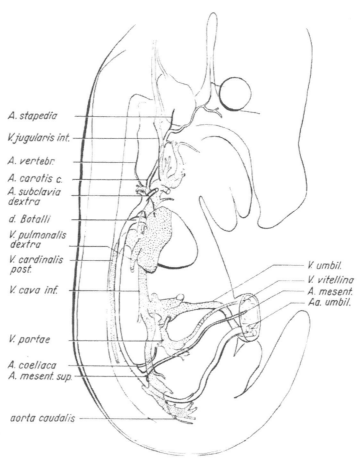

FIG. 224. Reconstruction of the vascular system, viewed from the right.
Stippled areas indicate venous system.
KT 643b, 14 days

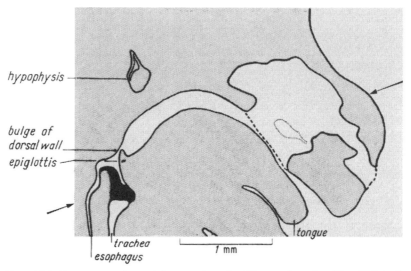

FIG. 225. Reconstruction of the nasal cavity. Plane of section Fig. 226 indicated by *arrows*. *Broken line* indicates communication within oral cavity. *Lightly stippled contour* indicates localization of Jacobson's organ, within the nasal septum.

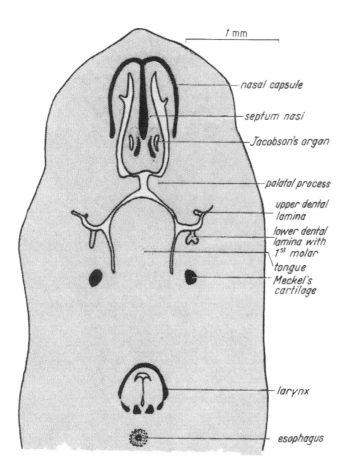

1 mm

- nasal capsule
- septum nasi
- Jacobson's organ
- palatal process
- upper dental lamina
- lower dental lamina with 1st molar
- tongue
- Meckel's cartilage
- larynx
- esophagus

FIG. 226. Transverse section of nasal cavities (for plane of section see Fig. 25, *arrows*).

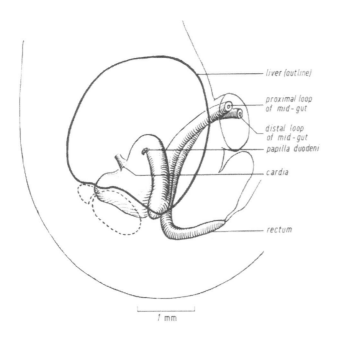

- liver (outline)
- proximal loop of mid-gut
- distal loop of mid-gut
- papilla duodeni
- cardia
- rectum

1 mm

FIG. 227. Reconstruction of mid- and hindgut, viewed from the right. *Dotted lines* indicate kidney and suprarenal.
KT 643b, 14 days

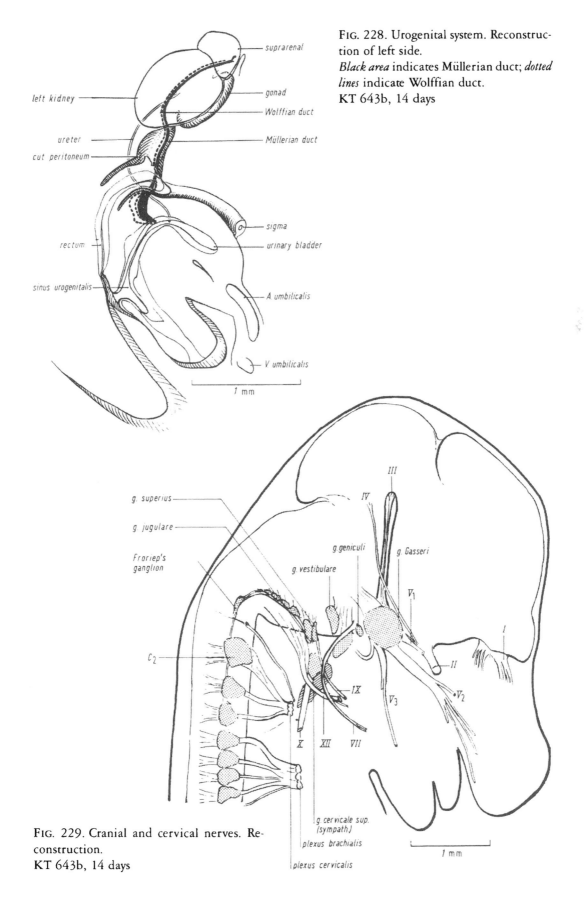

FIG. 228. Urogenital system. Reconstruction of left side.
Black area indicates Müllerian duct; *dotted lines* indicate Wolffian duct.
KT 643b, 14 days

suprarenal

gonad

Wolffian duct

Müllerian duct

left kidney

ureter

cut peritoneum

sigma

urinary bladder

rectum

A umbilicalis

sinus urogenitalis

V umbilicalis

1 mm

g. superius

g. jugulare

Froriep's ganglion

g. vestibulare

g. geniculi

g. Gasseri

III

IV

V_1

I

C_2

II

IX

V_3

V_2

X   XII   VII

g. cervicale sup. (sympath.)

plexus brachialis

plexus cervicalis

1 mm

FIG. 229. Cranial and cervical nerves. Reconstruction.
KT 643b, 14 days

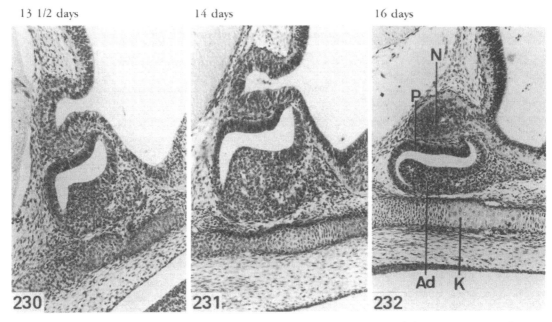

13 1/2 days   14 days   16 days

FIGS. 230–232. Development of hypophysis. Sagittal sections, 13 1/2–16 days (Figs. 230 and 231: 115:1. Fig. 232: 88:1).
K = cartilaginous base of skull (sphenoid), Ad = adenohypophysis, N = neurohypophysis, P = pars intermedia.

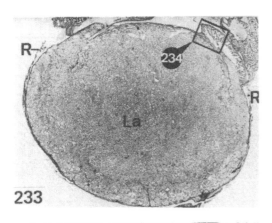

FIG. 233. Section of placenta, PAS-reaction.
La = labyrinth, R = Reichert's membrane.
KT 1017, 14 days 2 h. 12.5:1

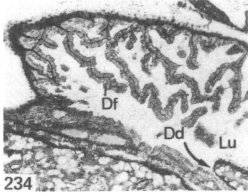

FIG. 234. Enlarged view.
Df = fold of yolk sac wall, Lu = lumen of yolk sac, Dd = "diverticle of yolk sac" (communication between lumen of yolk sac and intraplacental space).

Stage 23   Toes Separate
15 Days, 12–14 mm

Comparable to homo
2 months
(30–40 mm)

External Features

The most prominent feature to define this group is the separation of *toes* and "fingers" (Figs. 235 and 236). They are clearly divergent and will not become parallel until much later. The *pinna* covers more than half of the external auditory meatus. In the unfixed state, the superficial veins are often distinctly visible (Fig. 235).

In fixed specimens, the discrete elevations of the hair follicles may be seen all over the body. The eyelids are still open (Fig. 237). The 65 somites cannot be detected by external inspection.

Length. The length varies from 11.5 to 14 mm. In sagittal sections there are no important differences from the previous and the following stage.

Circulatory System

In the *heart*, the atrio-ventricular and semilunar valves are well developed. The stems of the coronary vessels are distinctly visible. The walls of the ventricles are smooth externally; internally, there are numerous indentations of small sinuses. The thickness of the wall is difficult to determine because the angle of section varies. The left ventricle seems to have a thicker wall than the right.

Arteries and *veins* now have the final fetal configuration, providing a larger umbilical circulation than yolk-sac circulation (Fig. 147). The details of the vascular system of this period will not be described.

Intestinal Tract

The oral and nasal cavities are completely separated by the palatal processes, which are now fusing with the nasal septum.

The *salivary glands* are distinct glandular trees. Most branches are solid epithelial cords leading to slender excretory ducts. The initial budding occurred at 12 days.

The enamel-organs of the incisors (Fig. 233, not labeled) are in an advanced stage of development. The newly arisen enamel organs of the first molars have a stellate reticulum (Fig. 226). The cartilage of the *larynx* and of the upper trachea is well developed.

The *thyroid* is subdivided into numerous small buds. Between these buds, abundant blood vessels can be observed. Follicles have not yet formed.

The *parathyroid* is now embedded in the thyroid. The ultimobranchial body is enclosed by thyroid tissue, and is said to give rise to the parafollicular cells.

The *thymus* can be recognized as a definite lymphatic organ. It is divided into lobules, which are not yet separated into medullary and cortical zones. In the center, there are many free lymphocytes. They are thought to be of mesenchymal rather than epithelial origin.

The *larynx* and *trachea* have a cartilaginous skeleton. The *lung* tissue is still rather compact, and it is more intensely vascularized than previously (compare Figs. 223 and 252).

Gut. Within the small intestine, numerous relatively thick villi have developed. In the large intestine, crypts are forming.

The *stomach* is distinctly separated into two parts. The glandular part has a tall columnar epithelium, which forms tiny folds. To the left, it is joined by the nonglandular portion, which has cuboidal and stratified epithelium. The musculature is arranged in several layers.

The *spleen* contains numerous blood vessels.

The *umbilical hernia* is still present.

Urogenital Tract

The *kidneys* contain centrally placed large glomeruli, with cuboidal perivascular cells. At the periphery of the organ, there is a wide zone of metanephric blastemal tissue, which borders the delicate capsule. Topographically, there is little change since 14 days (Fig. 228).

Sexual differentiation is greatly advanced.

The *ovary* has many dividing gonocytes, and they are often grouped in clusters.

In the *testis*, the solid seminiferous tubules are well differentiated. Near the surface, a condensation of cells forms the *tunica albuginea*. Diagnosis of sex is now very easy.

Central Nervous System

The *cortex* of the developing hemisphere is easily recognized at this stage. At the anterior boundary of the diencephalic roof, a small cellular area may be delimited, slightly anterior to the "Velum transversum" [158]. Some authors consider this cellular area to represent the paraphysis (Fig. 252, 16 days).

FIG. 235. Fetus of 14 days 23 h, 14 mm, life photograph. Distinct blood vessels.
KT 728. 4.7:1

FIG. 236. Different size in littermates of 14 days 20 h. Bouin fixation, 13.1 and 14.2 mm.
Nh = umbilical hernia.
KT 607 and 608. 4.5:1

FIG. 237. Eye, sagittal section, 14 days 23 h.
Lid = lower eyelid, *P* = pigmented layer, *C* = cornea, *G* = ganglion layer, *K* = nuclear layers.
KT 727. 105:1

FIG. 238. Hindfoot plate, 15 days 2 h.
Ti = tibia, *Ta* = talus, *Ca* = calcaneus, *Cu* = cuboid, *V* = metatarsale V.
KT 1030. 40.1

FIG. 239. Forefoot plate, 15 days 2 h.
Ra = radius, *Tr* = triquetrum, *Sc* = scaphoid-lunatum, *II.* = metacarpale II.
KT 1029. 40:1

FIG. 240. Radius, 15 days 2 h.
Ar = articulatio humero-radialis, *Ra* = radius.
KT 1029. 105:1

FIG. 241. Radius of Fig. 240 under high power.
K = periostal bone. 270:1

110

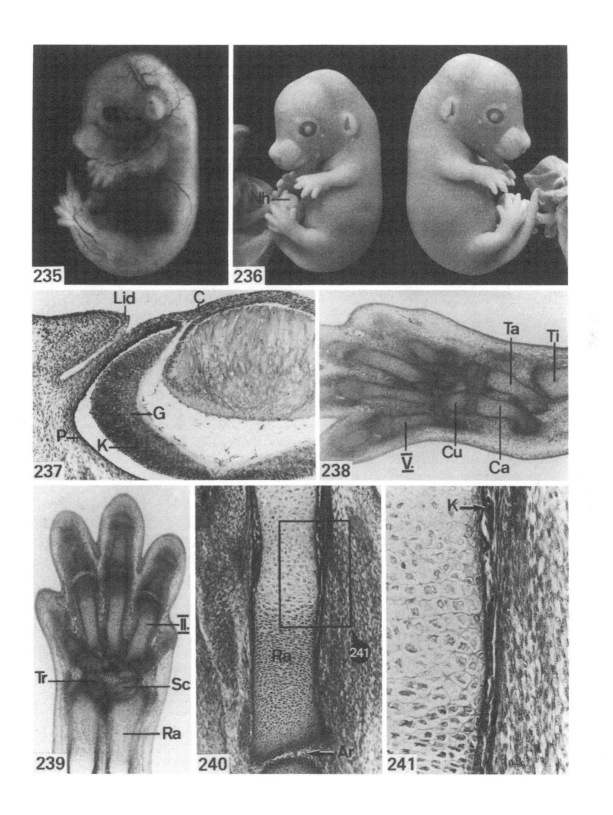

235

236

237   Lid   C
        G
    P   K

238   Ta   Ti
        Cu   Ca
        V.

239   II.
    Tr   Sc
        Ra

240   Ra   241
            Ar

241   K

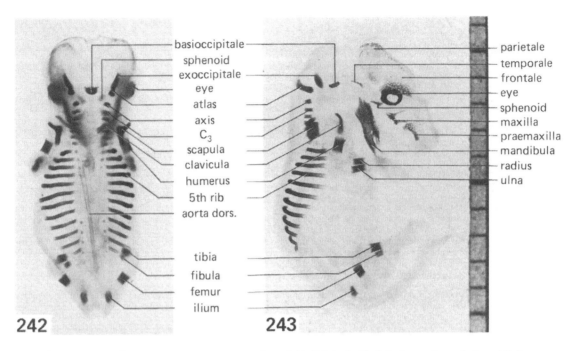

	basioccipitale		parietale
	sphenoid		temporale
	exoccipitale		frontale
	eye		eye
	atlas		sphenoid
	axis		maxilla
	C₃		praemaxilla
	scapula		mandibula
	clavicula		radius
	humerus		ulna
	5th rib		
	aorta dors.		
	tibia		
	fibula		
	femur		
242	ilium	**243**	

FIG. 242. Skeleton, dorsal view, 15 days 2 h. Alizarin-cleared preparation.
KT 1032

FIG. 243. Right half of skeleton, lateral view, 15 days 2 h.
Alizarin-cleared preparation.
KT 1032

The *hypophysis* is no longer connected to the pharyngeal roof (Figs. 231–232).

The *epiphysis* (Fig. 252, 16 days) acquires a lobular shape, but still has a central lumen.

The *eyelids* are more prominent (Fig. 237). The retina near the pupillary margin still has only one layer of cells. Located adjacent to the optic nerve, the ganglion cell layer may be distinguished from the undifferentiated nuclear layers.

Skeletal System

Alizarine-stained cleared preparations show many ossification centers; some of them having arisen during the preceding stage.

In the *skull*, ossification of the *os temporale* has just started, and it is easily identified in lateral view (Fig. 243).

Ossification centers of some vertebral arches are visible, but they have not yet appeared within the vertebral bodies (Fig. 242).

In the pelvic girdle, only the ossa ilii are stainable.

During this period, the long bones of the extremities show only periostal ossification in microscopic sections (Figs. 239–241).

Material	Age	
KT 727–28	14 days 23 h	6 embryos, 13.8–14 mm + 1 resorption
KT 1029–32	14 days 2 h	Several embryos from 11.5–12.5 mm

112

Stage 24   Reposition of Umbilical Hernia
16 Days, 14–17 mm

External Features

In the forefoot, *fingers* 2–5 are nearly parallel to each other, while the toes of the hindfoot still diverge. The *eyelids* have fused in most specimens. An epithelial mantle, a thin transparent membrane covering the cornea, is difficult to see by external inspection (Fig. 245). The external auditory meatus is almost completely covered by the *pinna*.

The *umbilical hernia* is disappearing, and the skin is becoming wrinkled.

The anterior part of the back is completely straight; this is more apparent than in 13–15 days embryos because of the increased length. In microscopic sections, however, the anterior vertebral column has a distinct lordotic curvature (Figs. 223 and 252).

Length. The length ranges, in extreme cases, between 14 and 18 mm.

Sagittal section (Fig. 252). The primary cortex of the *brain* is thickened and the choroid plexus is larger and divided into folds and villi.

The *abdominal cavity* has enlarged, so that the intestinal loops can be repositioned as the umbilical hernia is reduced.

Circulatory System

The heart and great vessels have the final prenatal configuration (Fig. 252).

The superficial veins are easily recognizable through the thin transparent skin (Figs. 245 and 246).

Intestinal Tract

A long slender *ductus nasopharyngeus* develops by further downward growth of the fused palatal processes. In this way, the epipharynx extends as far back as the prominent *epiglottis* (Fig. 252). The same sagittal section shows the anlage of the *incisors*.

The lip furrow (vestibulum oris) is still a solid plug of epithelial cells which will later split. The *thymus* increases strikingly in volume, surpassing considerably the neighboring thyroid (Fig. 252). The *thyroid* does not yet have follicles. Nevertheless, histologically it can be clearly distinguished from the parathyroids (Fig. 249).

The structure of the *lung* has not changed much since the previous stage.

The *stomach* is rapidly enlarging. The nonglandular portion, illustrated in Fig. 247, is lined by a multilayered cuboidal, sometimes flattened (squamous) epithelium.

The *spleen* (Fig. 247) contains distinct arteries and veins, separated by a rather compact tissue composed of various types of cells. Sometimes phagocytes can be recognized (Fig. 248), which seem to take up nuclei of red blood cells.

The *small intestine* now has longer, but still rather thick villi covered by columnar epithelium.

The large intestine is forming crypts.

In the *liver*, blood cell production is increasing. Externally, the final lobation is apparent [81]. The *pancreas* has finely branched, glandular trees, with distinct lumina, and pancreatic islets are budding. The typical β-cells cannot be seen with the light microscope until the 17th or 18th day [139].

The *suprarenals* appear as a regular network of strands composed of eosinophilic cells separated by wide capillaries. Scattered clusters of small medullary cells may also be seen.

Urogenital Tract

The *kidneys* still have a large peripheral metanephric blastema (Fig. 247). Near the center, many glomeruli are well developed.

In the *testes* distinct interstitial cells can now be recognized.

Central Nervous System

The primary cerebral cortex has enlarged considerably. In the diencephalon, the differentiation of the hypophysis and of the pineal gland is progressing. The epiphysis still has a central lumen, but the wall is markedly thickened (in Fig. 252 the wall is sectioned tangentially).

FIG. 244. Eye, horizontal section, 16 days, 15 mm.
Lid = lower eyelid, *C* = cornea, *L* = lens, *G* = ganglion layer of retina.
KT 646. 105:1

FIG. 245. Fetus of 16 days, life photograph, 15 mm.
KT 646

FIG. 246. Diagram of Fig. 245.
V.u. = vena umbilicalis, *V. v.* = vena vitellina, *Nh* = umbilical hernia (partially repositioned), *P* = placenta, *O* = pinna, *V.t.* = vena temporalis superficialis, *V.c.* = vena cephalica, *V.th.* = vena thoracica lateralis, *V.m.* = venae metatarseae dorsales.

FIG. 247. Cross section, at the level of the spleen, 16 days.
Ma = stomach, *Md* = mesogastrium dorsale, *Ni* = left kidney, *RM* = spinal cord, *Ar* = rudiment of vertebral articulation.
KT 646. 40:1

FIG. 248. Enlarged view of spleen in Fig. 247, with phagocyte (*arrow*) containing presumably nuclei of erythroblasts.
A = artery. 550:1

FIG. 249. Cross section, level of larynx, 16 days.
Ly = lymph vessel, *X* = nervus vagus, *Vj* = vena jugularis interna, *Ac* = arteria carotis communis, *Th* = thyreoidea (thyroid gland), *Pt* = parathyroid, *S* = cartilago thyreoidea, *La* = cavum laryngis.
KT 646. 105:1

FIG. 250. Sagittal section through 5th thoracic vertebra.
RM = spinal cord, *Ch* = notochordal segment, *Cs* = notochordal sheath, situated dorsally in calcified center of cartilage.
KT 646. 15 days. 105:1

FIG. 251. Sagittal section through axis, 16 days.
Cs = notochordal sheath, on clivus; *A* = anterior arch of atlas; *Af* = anulus fibrosus; *C3* = body of 3rd cervical vertebra.
KT 646. 105:1

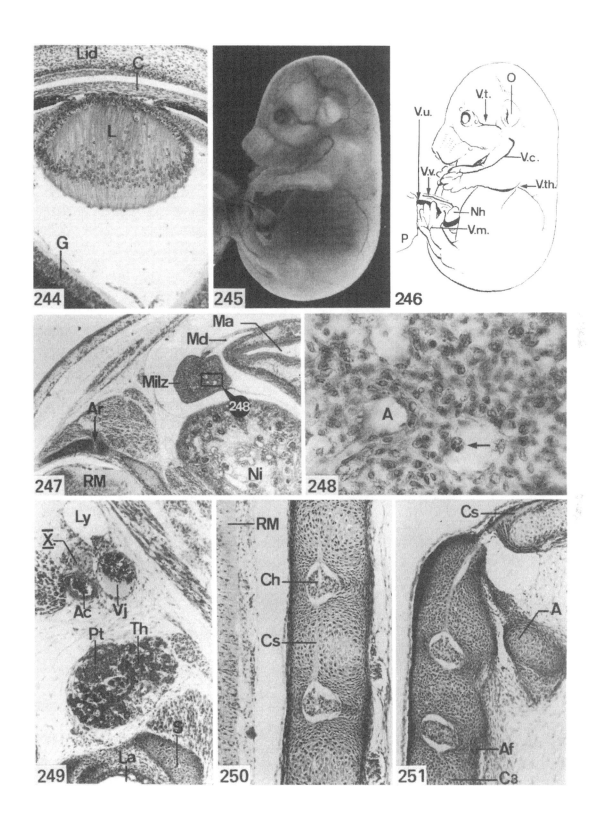

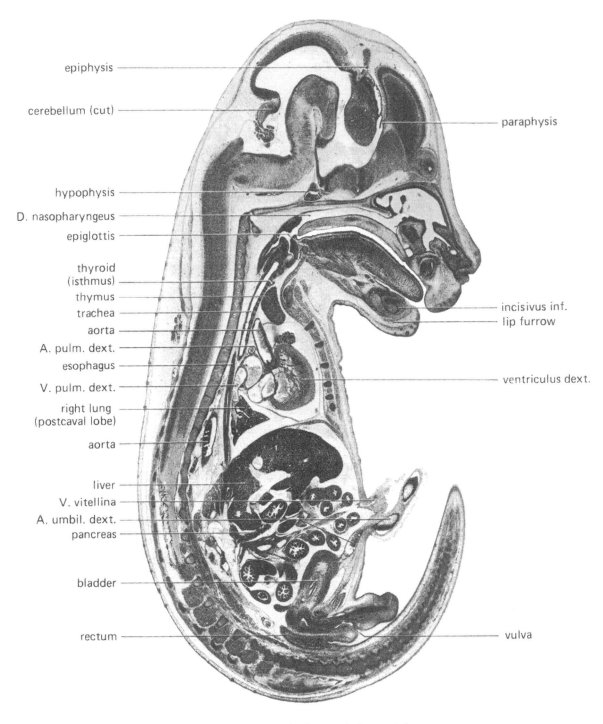

epiphysis

cerebellum (cut)

paraphysis

hypophysis

D. nasopharyngeus

epiglottis

thyroid (isthmus)

thymus

trachea

aorta

A. pulm. dext.

esophagus

V. pulm. dext.

right lung (postcaval lobe)

aorta

liver

V. vitellina

A. umbil. dext.

pancreas

bladder

rectum

incisivus inf.

lip furrow

ventriculus dext.

vulva

FIG. 252. Sagittal section. Female fetus, 16 days, 14.6 mm.
KT 646

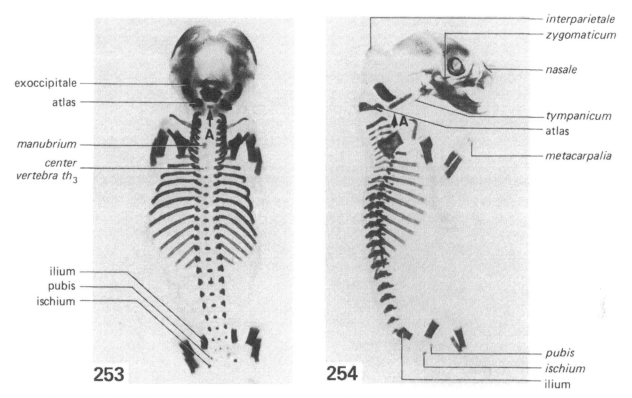

exoccipitale
atlas
manubrium
*center
vertebra th₃*
ilium
pubis
ischium

interparietale
zygomaticum
nasale
tympanicum
atlas
metacarpalia
pubis
ischium
ilium

253 **254**

FIGS. 253–254. Alizarin-cleared preparations. Fetuses of 16 days. *New skeletal elements in italics* (in the previous stage, Figs. 242–243, these were not yet visible). *Arrows* indicate ossification center of anterior arch of atlas.

Anterior to the velum transversum, a small area represents the parphysis (Graumann [158]).

A thin transparent epithelial membrane is growing over the cornea of the *eye*. The iris and the corpus ciliare cannot yet be distinguished. The anterior chamber of the eye extends beyond the pupillary margin (Fig. 244).

The *retina* is not much more differentiated than in the 15-day stage. The labyrinth has a well developed cartilaginous capsule, which encloses the semicircular ducts and the ductus cochlearis. The sensory epithelia are thickened, but not well differentiated.

Skeletal System

Most of the vertebral bodies contain initial ossification centers, i.e., calcium deposits within the cartilage, as shown in Fig. 250. Photographs of sagittal sections through the fifth thoracic vertebra will illustrate, in later stages, progressing ossification.

A salient feature of this developmental stage is the appearance of ossification centers in the anterior arch of the atlas and in other skeletal elements whose labels are in italics in Figs. 253–254.

Material	Age	
KT 646–47	16 days 2 h	7 fetuses, 14.0–15.2 mm
KT 1046–48	16 days 4 h	5 fetuses, 16–18 mm + 1 resorption

Stage 25 Fingers and Toes Joined Together
17 Days, 17–20 mm

External Features
The skin is wrinkled and thickened, and the subcutaneous veins are no longer distinctly visible (compare Figs. 256 and 245). The eyelids are fused and thickened. The fingers and toes are parallel. In all cases examined, the umbilical hernia has disappeared.

Length. There is considerable variation in length due to different degrees of curvature of the fetuses: 16.5–20 mm in the unfixed state.

Circulatory System
The pattern of the superficial veins has not changed since the previous stage, but is more difficult to recognize.

Intestinal Tract
The shape of the oral and nasal cavities has not changed much.

Endocrine derivatives. The *thyroid* is a bilobed organ, with a narrow isthmus. The solid, branched epithelial cords are beginning to form small well-vascularized follicles.

The *parathyroids* are forming compact clusters of cells on each side, which join the posterior margins of the thyroid lobes.

FIG. 255. Living fetus, frontal view, 17 days, 20 mm.
KT 908

FIG. 256. Living fetus, viewed from the left, 17 days, 20 mm.
KT 908

FIG. 257. Living fetus, viewed from the right. Same developmental stage, but one day older, 18 days, 20 mm.
KT 657. 4:1

FIG. 258. Eye, horizontal section, enlarged view of Fig. 260.
C = cornea, I = iris rudiment, Cc = corpus ciliare, G = ganglion layer of retina, Pl = punctum lacrimale (on inner surface of eyelid).
KT 724, 17 days. 105:1

FIG. 259. Pineal gland, sagittal section, 17 days.
V = vena cerebri interna.
KT 724. 105:1

FIG. 260. Low power view of eye, with nervus opticus and vicinity.
K = caput mandibulae, gG = ganglion Gasseri, N = nasal cavity.
KT 724, 17 days. 27:1

FIG. 261. Sagittal section through thoracic vertebrae 4 and 5 (Th_4 and Th_5) +/+ fetus, 17 days.
Cs = notochord sheath, D = dura mater spinalis. 105:1

FIG. 262. Sagittal section through axis, 17 days.
A = anterior arch of atlas, Af = anulus fibrosus C_2/C_3, Lt = ligamentum transversum atlantis, Cs = notochord sheath.
KT 908. 100:1

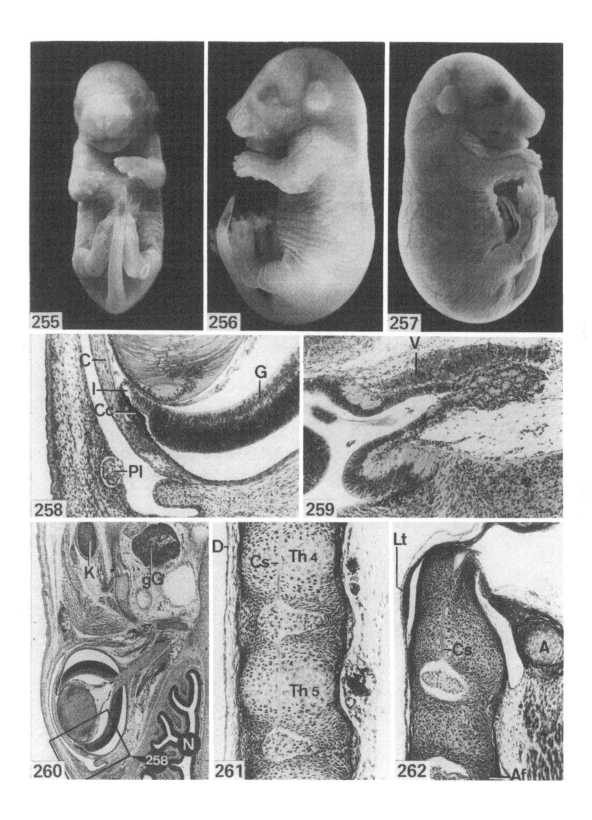

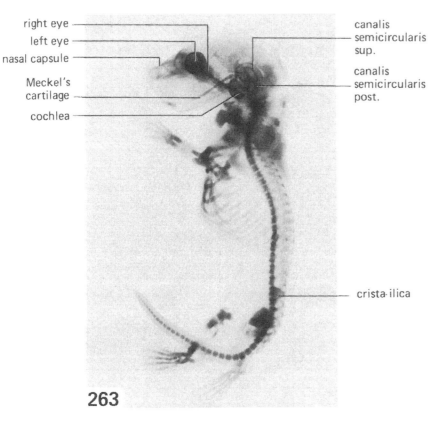

right eye
left eye
nasal capsule
Meckel's cartilage
cochlea

canalis semicircularis sup.
canalis semicircularis post.

FIG. 263. Cartilaginous skeleton with 17 days. Cleared preparation, methylgreen. KT 776

FIG. 264. Alizarin cleared preparation, 17 days 23 h. Dorsal view. *New bones in italics. A (arrow)* indicates ossification center in anterior arch of atlas. KT 1028

crista·ilica

FIG. 265. Right half of skeleton, same specimen as shown in Fig. 264.

263

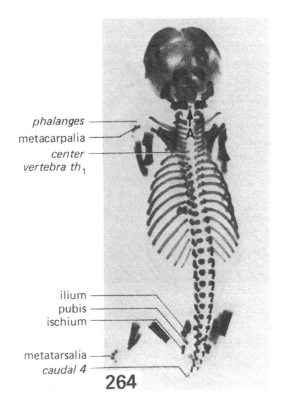

phalanges
metacarpalia
center vertebra th₁

ilium
pubis
ischium

metatarsalia
caudal 4

264

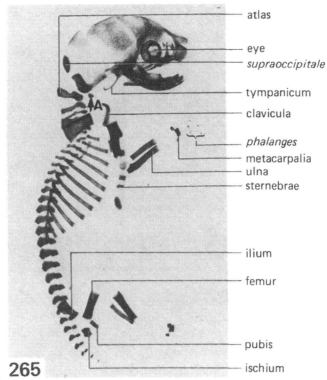

atlas
eye
supraoccipitale
tympanicum
clavicula
phalanges
metacarpalia
ulna
sternebrae

ilium
femur

pubis

ischium

265

The *thymus* is now a large organ, separated into two bilaterally situated main lobes containing numerous small blood vessels. Sometimes aggregations of reticulum may be seen, but there are no Hassal's corpuscles.

The structure of the *lungs* appears less compact now.

The respiratory pathways are extending peripherally.

The developing aveolar ducts are lined by cuboidal epithelium.

The *intestines* are quite similar to the previous stage.

The *spleen* is elongating rapidly. It contains, for the first time, lymphocytes.

The *adrenal glands* have a more continuous medullary region consisting of small pale cells, which differ sharply from the large, intensively stained cells of the cortex.

The *testes* have well formed tunicae albugineae. Numerous scattered interstitial cells are recognizable singly or in groups.

The *ovaries* contain many oocytes, often grouped together. They have entered the meiotic prophase.

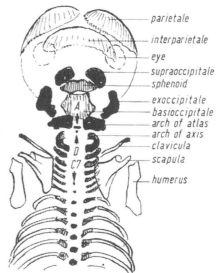

FIG. 266. Dorsal view of alizarin cleared preparation, cranial part, 17 days.

D = ossification center in basis of dens, newly arisen; A = anterior arch of atlas; C7 = ossification center in body of 7th cervical vertebra.

KT 1028

Central Nervous System

Because of the gland-like budding of its epithelium (Fig. 259), the distal part of the lumen of the epiphysis is disappearing.

The eyelids are closed. The ciliary body is delineated (Fig. 258).

The capsule of the *labyrinth* has assumed its definite shape (Fig. 263).

Skeletal System

The skeletal system is best studied in cleared specimens (Figs. 264 and 265). Labels of new bones, which now stain with alizarin red S, are in italics in the legend, i.e., phalanges, etc. It should be pointed out that calcified cartilage may also be stained, and microscopically it is different from bone. Histologic sections of some vertebrae are illustrated in Figs. 261 and 262.

The ossification of the vertebral bodies begins in the lower thoracic region and has now proceeded forward to the first thoracic vertebra. The anterior arch of the atlas has already begun to ossify, and the basal ossification center of the dens is also developing at this early stage. The centrum of the dens axis is just appearing (Fig. 266). The centrum of the axis body will appear soon.

Material	Age	
KT 724–25	17 days	8 fetuses, 17–17.5 mm
KT 908	17 days	3 fetuses, 18–20 mm
KT 1052	17 days 2 h	8 fetuses, 18–20 mm
KT 1049–50	17 days 3 h	7 fetuses, 16.5–19.5 mm

121

Stage 26   Long Whiskers
18 Days, 19.5–22.5 mm

External Features

The whiskers, visible at 17 days as short filaments (Fig. 255), are now definitely longer. The skin is thickened and markedly wrinkled. The eyes are barely visible through the closed eyelids.

Length. Because of different degrees of curvature, the length varies from 18 to 23 mm.

Circulatory System

The final prenatal configuration of the circulation system was established at 16–17 days.

Intestinal Tract

In the *oral cavity*, the rate of development of the first molars is remarkable. The stellate reticulum is enlarged and the outer enamel organ epithelium is in close contact with numerous capillaries. The ameloblastic layer, composed of tall cylindrical cells, has the form of the future crown. In Fig. 270, the enamel organ is separated from the surrounding loose connective tissue by artificial shrinkage. The second molar is about 2 days later in development than the first.

Derivatives of the Intestinal Tract

In the *thyroid* the number of colloid-filled follicles has increased considerably. Between the numerous lobuli, there is loose connective tissue containing many blood vessels. The secretory activity seems to be intensive.

Both *parathyroids* may be recognized as rather compact, spherical cell clusters, closely adhered to the thyroid. They are situated on each side somewhat below the middle of the lobes. Many blood vessels have grown between the parenchymal cords.

The *pancreatic islands* are now well differentiated.

The *thymus* has enlarged further (Fig. 275). There is no clear boundary between the medulla and cortex. In the medulla, extensive aggregations of large clear reticulum cells are visible. There are numerous blood vessels.

Respiratory System

The structure of the *lungs* has changed completely: one could speak of an "alveolar explosion." There is a sudden development of large alveolar ducts and of sac-like primitive alveoli lined by cuboidal epithelium. The resulting loose structure of the lung tissue is visible with low magnification.

The *larynx* and *trachea* have completed their prenatal differentiation.

Abdominal Viscera

There have been no marked changes in the abdominal viscera since the preceding stage. The *spleen* has elongated, is rich in cells, and exhibits signs of intensive blood formation.

There is still active hemopoiesis in the *liver*.

In the *stomach*, the subdivision into glandular and nonglandular part is clearly visible. In the *gut*, the characteristic relief of the lining has developed.

Urogenital Tract

The *kidneys* are about the same as in the preceding age group.

The *glands* of the male genital excretory ducts are now very conspicuous, and the *seminal vesicles* (Fig. 275) contain distinct lumina. The lumen of the bulbo-urethral gland (Cowper's gland) is just forming and it opens into the urethra together with the recessus bulbosus.

The *prostate gland* is appearing as short, solid cords of epithelial cells budding from the pars prostatica urethrae.

The tunica albuginea of the *testis* has increased in thickness. The seminiferous tubules are still solid and are connected with the canalicular system of the rete testis (Fig. 276). The gonocytes have stopped dividing [118]. Between the tubuli contorti, there are numerous interstitial cells.

Ovaries (Figs. 278 and 279). The ovaries are closely attached to the lower poles of the kidneys. The bursa ovarica almost completely surrounds the ovary. In the mesosalpinx, many mesonephric tubules can be recognized. Some oocytes are being encircled by flat epithelial cells, which form the *primary follicles*.

Central Nervous System

The rudiment of the *pineal gland* has been transformed into a stalked, glandular organ.

Within the *hypophysis*, the original lumen of Rathke's pouch is narrowed (Fig. 271). The adenohypophysis assumes the appearance of a typical endocrine gland.

In the *brain*, the olfactory lobe is well developed.

In the *eye*, the iris and corpus ciliare are well formed (Fig. 272).

Skeletal System

Skull. The bilaterally situated ossification centers of the supraoccipitale have fused (compare Figs. 281 and 266).

Vertebral column. The vertebral bodies C_2-C_5 still lack ossification centers.

Extremities. Ossification of the extremities is proceeding rapidly (Fig. 280).

Adipose tissue is abundant in the subcutaneous tissue of the neck. It probably is a source of energy for the postnatal period, and has been called "multilocular adipose tissue" (MAT, Fig. 275).

Material	Age	
KT 656–57	17 days 21 h	5 fetuses, 18.5–20.5 mm
KT 1010–11	17 days 23 h	6 fetuses, 18.0–20.0 mm
KT 1023–28	17 days 23 h	6 fetuses, 19.0–21.0– mm
KT 1041–42	18 days 4 h	6 fetuses, 23 mm

FIG. 267. Fetus of 17 days 23 h, 22.2 mm. Formalin fixation.
KT 1027

FIG. 268. Same fetus viewed from the right. 3:1

FIG. 269. Alizarin-cleared preparation, 17 days 23 h.
For explanation, see Fig. 280.
KT 1011. 3.5:1

FIG. 270. Cross section through head, level of eyes, 17 days 23 h.
CN = cavum nasi, *DN* = ductus naso-pharyngeus (compare Figs. 252 and 225), *Olf* = lobus olfactorius, *Sp* = stellate reticulum (molar). 23:1

FIG. 271. Hypophysis, sagittal section, 18 days 4 h.
N = neurohypophysis (posterior lobe), *P* = pars intermedia, *Ad* = adenohypophysis (anterior lobe), *T* = pars tuberalis.
KT 1041/3. 130:1

FIG. 272. Enlarged view of eye in Fig. 270.
Cc = corpus ciliare, *I* = iris, *Ln* = suture of eyelids. 60:1

FIG. 273. Sagittal section through 5th thoracic vertebra, 18 days 4 h.
Cs = notochordal sheath, *P* = periostal bone, ventral part.
KT 1041/3. 105:1

FIG. 274. Sagittal section through axis, 17 days 23 h.
A = arcus anterior atlantis, *D* = dura mater cerebri (above clivus), *De* = ossification center in basis of dens, *C3* = body of 3rd cervical vertebra.
KT 1010. 55:1

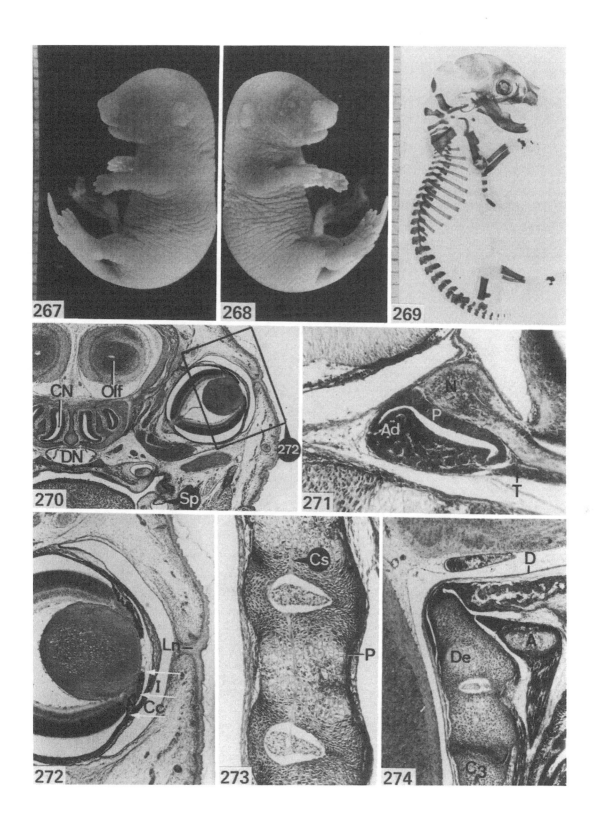

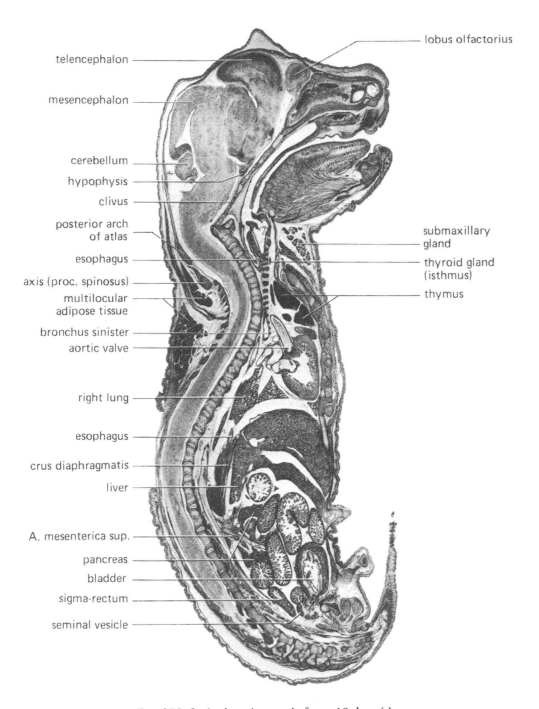

telencephalon

mesencephalon

cerebellum

hypophysis

clivus

posterior arch
of atlas

esophagus

axis (proc. spinosus)

multilocular
adipose tissue

bronchus sinister

aortic valve

right lung

esophagus

crus diaphragmatis

liver

A. mesenterica sup.

pancreas

bladder

sigma-rectum

seminal vesicle

lobus olfactorius

submaxillary
gland

thyroid gland
(isthmus)

thymus

FIG. 275. Sagittal section, male fetus, 18 days 4 h,
23 mm.
KT 1041

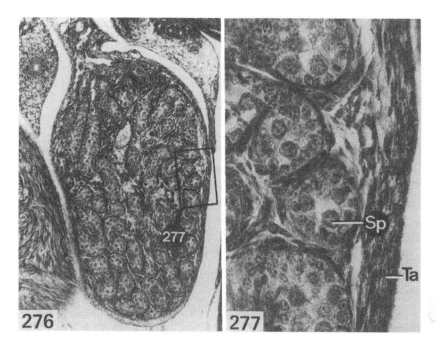

FIG. 276. Sagittal section through
testis, 17 days 23 h.
KT 1010. 105:1

FIG. 277. High power view of testis
Fig. 276.
Sp = spermatogonium, *Ta* = tunica
albuginea. 550:1

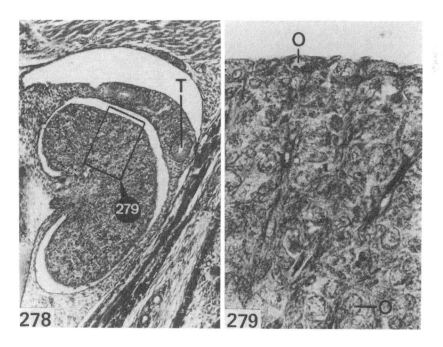

FIG. 278. Ovary, frontal section,
17 days 23 h.
T = oviduct.
KT 1010/30. 105:1

FIG. 279. High power view of ovary
Fig. 278.
0 = oocytes. 550:1

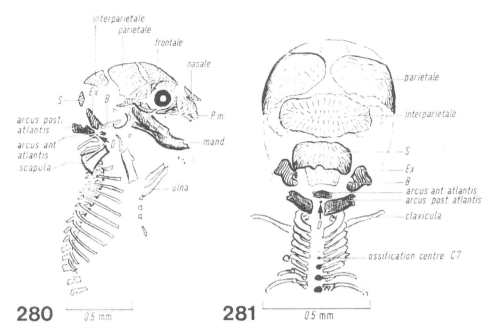

280   0.5 mm   281   0.5 mm

FIGS. 280–281. Alizarin-cleared preparations, 18 days, 22 m. Anterior part of the body in lateral (Fig. 280) and dorsal view (Fig. 281).

B = basioccipitale, *Ex* = exoccipitale, *S* = supraoccipitale, *D* (*arrow*) = ossification center in basis of dens, *P.m.* = premaxilla.

KT 1011

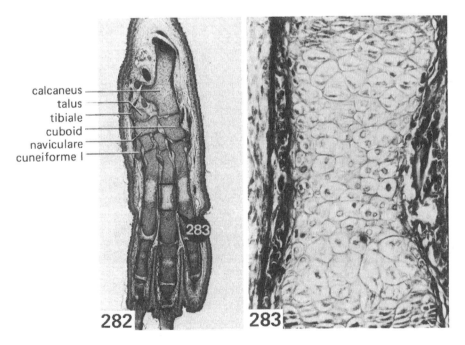

FIG. 282. Horizontal section through hind-foot plate, 17 days 23 h.
KT 1026. 22:1

FIG. 283. Enlarged view of metatarsale 3 (Fig. 282).
270:1

Stage 27 Newborn Mouse
19 Days, 23–27 mm.

External Features

The external appearance of the newborn mouse is not essentially different from the preceding stage (18 days), but the animal is considerably longer. The eyes and ears have closed. Histologically they are quite immature. The pigmented eye is still visible through the skin, which is thicker than in the 18-day fetus. The dark shadows of the liver and of the spleen (on the left side) can be seen through the body wall and the skin. Milk in the stomach can also be seen externally. The whiskers are long and clearly visible. The hair does not appear until the mouse is 2 or 3 days old.

The vagina remains closed for more than one month after birth.

Length. There is considerable variation in length, mainly due to different degrees of flexure of the body axis. Living newborns are usually 23 to 27 mm, but a few may be longer.

Circulatory System

The *ductus Botalli* (Fig. 293) has a tiny lumen for several hours after birth.

The blood vessels of the lungs are considerably distended.

The foramen ovale (Fig. 294) is anatomically open, but functionally closed.

Near their entrance into the heart, the veins have distinct valves, i.e., at the termination of the vena jugularis externa, interna, and at the inlet of the caval veins into the atrium (Fig. 294).

Intestinal Tract

The *oral cavity* has long been completely separated from the nasal cavities (Fig. 292).

The primordia of the incisors are shown in Fig. 292. The dental papilla (marked by the end of the line in Fig. 292) is bordered by tall odontoblasts. They already have formed some predentine. Peripherally, a layer of tall ameloblasts can be seen.

Derivatives of the Intestinal Tract

The *thyroid* (Fig. 295) is actively secreting. There are only two *parathyroids* in the mouse and they are bilaterally attached to the thyroid lobes. Displaced clusters of parathyroid cells are occasionally found within the connective tissue septa of the thymus [143].

The cortex of the *thymus* (Fig. 296) is subdivided into two zones:

1. an outer zone, containing large lymphoid cells, some of them in mitosis, and
2. an inner zone, with many small lymphocytes.

In the medulla there are clusters of large clear reticulum cells. Hassal's corpuscles are lacking.

FIG. 284. Newborn mouse, from the left, 27 mm.
L = liver, Sp = spleen, M = stomach (filled with milk). 2.5:1

FIG. 285. Same specimens as in Fig. 284, right side, with millimeter scale. 2.5:1

FIG. 286. Alizarin-cleared preparation, newborn.
S = supraoccipitale, A = arcus posterior atlantis, Sc = scapula dextra, OJ = os ilii, F = femur, TC = talus and calcaneus.
KT 891. 2.2:1

FIG. 287. First picture of dissection, newborn mouse.
T = thymus; H = heart, in pericardium; Pc = lobus postcavalis of right lung; L = liver; B = bladder, filled. 2.5:1

FIG. 288. Second picture of dissection, same newborn mouse. Sm = glandula submaxillaris, T = thymus, P = pancreas, M = stomach, Sp = spleen, Si = colon sigmoideum, N = left kidney, C = cecum, J = ileum. 2.5:1

FIG. 289. Sagittal section through 4th and 5th thoracic vertebra, 19 days.
Cs = notochordal sheath, D = dura mater. 90:1

FIG. 290. Eye, frontal section, newborn mouse.
O = nervus opticus, Ln = suture of eye lids, G = ganglion cell layer.
KT 1067. 55:1

FIG. 291. High power view of iris (Fig. 290).
I = iris, Cc = corpus ciliate, Mi = mitosis in lens epithelium. 270:1

130

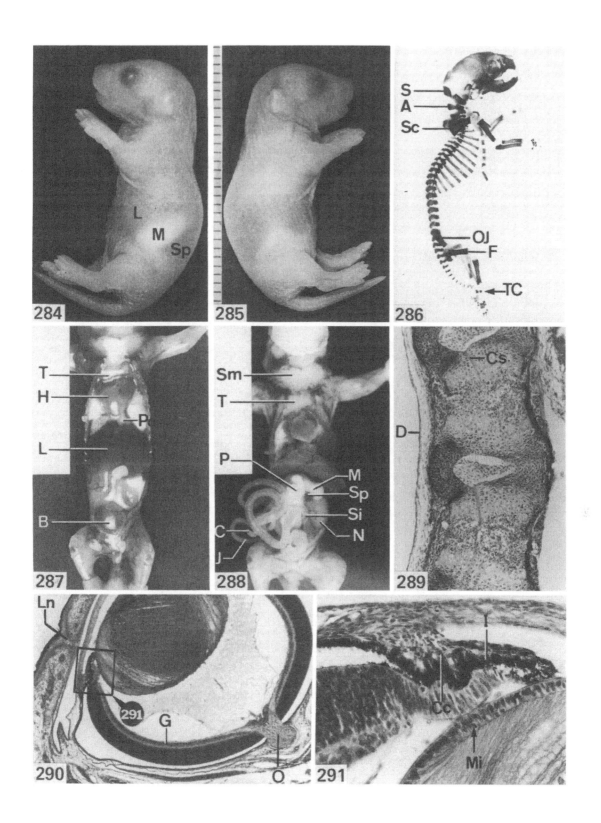

Respiratory System

The left *lung* consists of one undivided lobe. The right lung is subdivided into 4 lobes. In addition to the upper-, middle-, and lower lobes there is a special lobus postcavalis. It is behind the heart, and extends quite far into the left side of the body (Fig. 294). Each bronchus lobaris gives off regular segmental and subsegmental bronchi (Fig. 301). The latter are connected to short terminal bronchi, which open into wide alveolar sacs. There is a gradual transition between the cuboidal epithelium of the terminal bronchi and the flattened cells lining the aveoli. Except for the stem bronchi, the bronchial walls of the mouse do not contain cartilage.

Abdominal Viscera

The *liver* and *spleen* are sites of active hemopoiesis. The most conspicuous type of hemopoietic cells is the megakaryocyte and it is found in both organs. In the spleen, a few nodules of lymphatic tissue have formed. These are more distinct after birth [57].

The *stomach* is relatively large. It shows signs of marked secretory activity. The duodenum is the widest part of the intestine, and it has numerous villi. The large intestine is of the same caliber as the small intestine (Fig. 292).

The *adrenal glands* (Fig. 292) are well developed. The cortex and medulla are now more distinctly demarcated than at 17 days (Fig. 298). The medullary cells are smaller than the cortical cells.

In the cortex, three zones may be distinguished (Fig. 298):

1. a narrow outer zone, composed of small, crowded cells.
2. a large middle zone, consisting of large cells with abundant cytoplasm in which vacuoles (dissolved lipids) can be seen sometimes. The cells are not arranged in parallel strands; and
3. a narrow inner zone with small, intensively stained cells. They are the precursors of the X-zone, which will develop after birth. It will regress at the age of one month.

In the medulla, the peripheral cells (bordering the cortex) are often clustered together, reflecting their original arrangement in small groups. Between them there are intensively stained strands of cortical cells. The clusters of young medullary cells should not be confused with hemopoietic foci. Their nuclei are larger and lighter than erythroblastic nuclei, and their cytoplasm is basophilic.

Urogenital Tract

There is a wide peripherally situated growth zone in the kidneys.

Diagnosis of sex. The perineum is definitely longer in the male. The distance between anus and genital papilla in the female is roughly one-half that in the male.

The topography of the *internal genital organs* is shown in simplified form in sketches of reconstructions (Figs. 303 and 304). The large seminal vesicle opens into a common orifice with the ampulla ductus deferentis into the urethra, at the colliculus seminalis. Later, a separate opening is often observed. The coagulating gland can be seen as a short sprout, situated immediately anterior (proximal) to the colliculus seminalis (Fig. 303). Other sprouts visible in Fig. 303 are primordia of the prostate (not labeled).

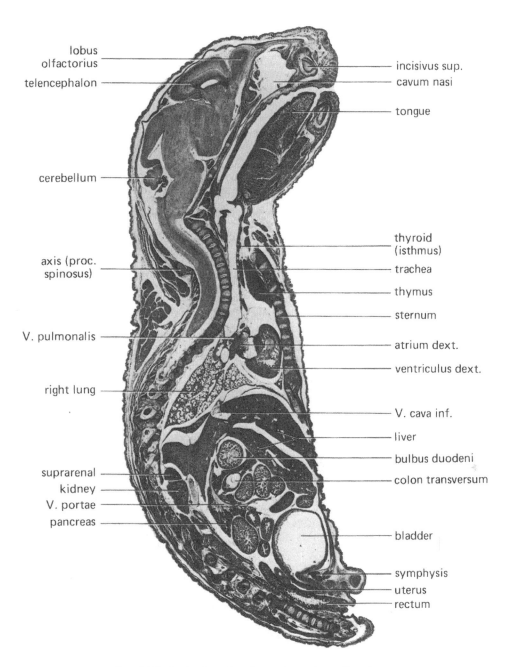

lobus olfactorius
telencephalon
cerebellum
axis (proc. spinosus)
V. pulmonalis
right lung
suprarenal
kidney
V. portae
pancreas

incisivus sup.
cavum nasi
tongue
thyroid (isthmus)
trachea
thymus
sternum
atrium dext.
ventriculus dext.
V. cava inf.
liver
bulbus duodeni
colon transversum
bladder
symphysis
uterus
rectum

FIG. 292. Sagittal section through newborn female mouse.
KT 1067

133

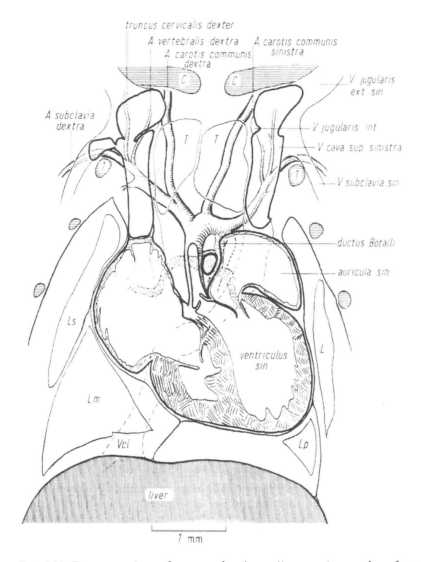

FIG. 293. Reconstructions of aorta and pulmonalis, superimposed on frontal section, ventral view.

Pulmonalis and ductus Botalli indicated by *stippled areas*; contours of large veins are indicated. *C* = clavicula, *1* = costa 1, *T* = thymus, *L* = left lung, *Lp* = lobus superior postcavalis (pulmonis dextri), *Lm* = lobus medius, *Ls* = lobus superior, *Vci* = vena cava inferior (projection).

KT 1067, newborn

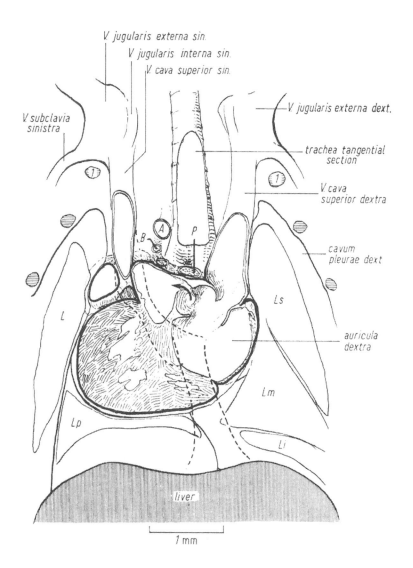

FIG. 294. Reconstruction of venous inlet, superimposed on frontal section. Dorsal view. *Broken lines* indicate course of caval veins. *A* = arcus aortae, *P* = arteria pulmonalis dextra, *B* = ductus Botalli, *L* = left lung, *Ls* = lobus superior, *Lm* = lobus medius, *Li* = lobus inferior, *Lp* = lobus postcavalis. *Arrow* indicates foramen ovale. KT 1067

FIG. 295. Thyroid isthmus, newborn mouse.
F = follicle. 550:1

FIG. 296. Thymus, newborn mouse.
Arrow indicates mitosis of a lymphoblast. 550:1

FIG. 297. Liver, newborn mouse.
Me = megakaryocyte, *P* = branch of portal vein. 270:1

FIG. 298. Suprarenals, low power view, newborn mouse. 220:1

FIG. 299. High power view of boundary zone cortex–medulla (Fig. 298). 550:1

FIG. 300. Pancreas, newborn mouse.
In = pancreatic island.
KT 910. 550:1

FIG. 301. Frontal section through left lung, newborn mouse.
KT 1067. 40:1

FIG. 302. High power view of lung subsegment.
Sa = saccus alveolaris. 270:1

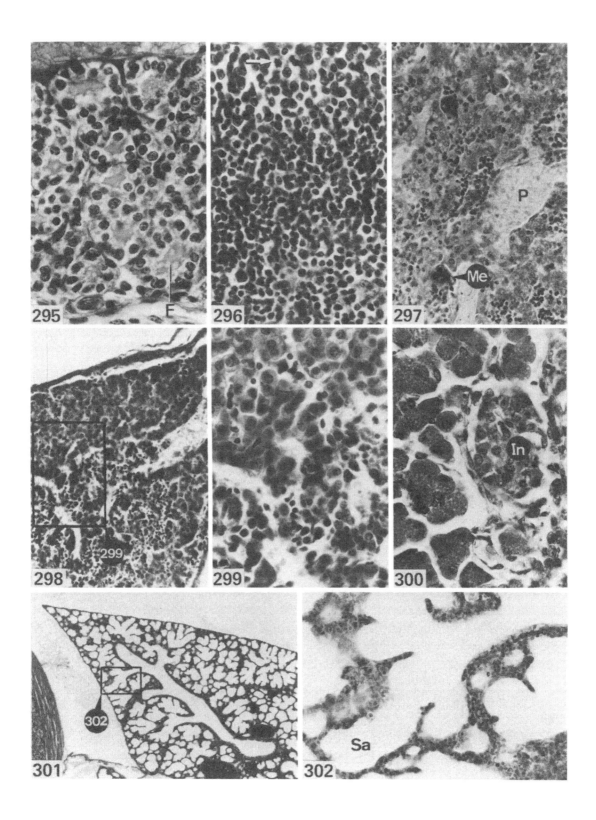

295

296

297 P Me

298 299

299 300 In

301 302

302 Sa

137

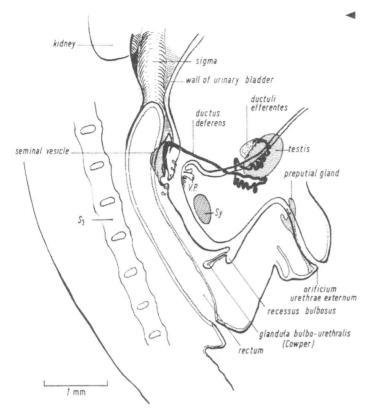

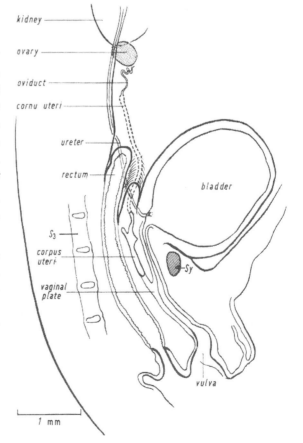

FIG. 303. Male genital organs. Reconstruction, newborn mouse. Left half, viewed from the right.
Caput and cauda epididymidis shown in simplified form. *V.P.* = ventral prostat, Sy = symphysis, S_3 = 3rd sacral vertebra.
KT 910

FIG. 304. Female genital organs. Reconstruction, newborn mouse. Left half, viewed from the right.
Oviduct shown in simplified form. Sy = symphysis.
KT 1067

In the *ovary* many cells with condensed chromosomes can be seen, mostly prophases of the first meiotic division of the oocytes. Some primary follicles have developed in the more central area of the ovary. In this region, the oocytes are in the dictyotene stage. Graafian follicles are absent. The surface of the ovary is exposed to the fluid-filled space of the bursa ovarica, which is almost completely closed [107].

In the *testis* there are many interstitial cells. The tubuli contorti are composed of numerous primitive Sertoli cells (nourishing and supporting cells) and large gonocytes (Fig. 305). The *gonocytes* are no longer dividing. Mitotic activity will be resumed during the first week after birth. Simultaneously, the gonocytes will migrate toward the basement membrane of the seminiferous tubules. The developing daughter cells will be

138

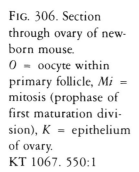
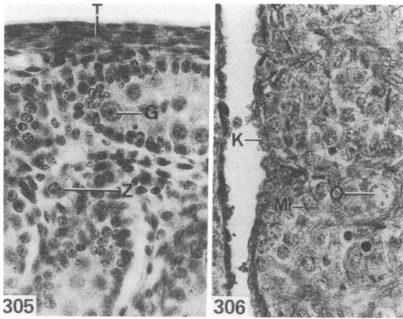

smaller and are called immature spermatogonia type A. Mature spermatogonia will remain smaller. These cells are generally flattened and closely attached to the basement membrane. They appear at the initiation of spermatogenesis.

Central Nervous System

In the *cerebellum*, the fissures that developed in the previous stage have deepened considerably (Fig. 292). The structure of the hypophysis [136], which can be used as an indication of developmental age, has not changed, compared with Fig. 271 (18 days).

The accessory organs of the *eye* have appeared. The conductory system of the infraorbital gland is composed of numerous branches. The passage opens into the saccus conjunctivae, together with the neighboring solid sprouts of the lacrimal gland. The Harderian gland reaches the conjunctiva by a single, slender duct, in the neighborhood of the nicticating membrane. These glands are not differentiated histologically. The nicticating membrane, however, contains some cartilage.

The iris and corpus ciliare (Fig. 291) remain at the state of maturation attained one day earlier (18 days, Fig. 272).

The *internal ear* is only slightly changed since day 18. The external auditory meatus has closed. The auditory apparatus cannot function until the second week after birth, when the organ of Corti has completed its maturation [180].

Skeletal System

The *vertebral column* has changed between the stage of 18 days and the newborn, but the skull remains about the same. All ossification centers of the vertebral bodies of the trunk have formed, including cervical 3–5 (compare Fig. 307 to Figs. 280 and 281). Ossification is well advanced in the thoracic region (Fig. 289).

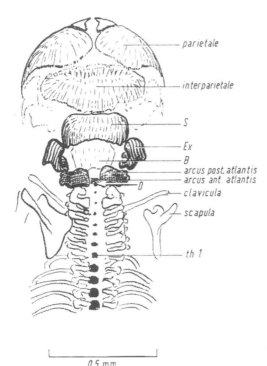

FIG. 307. Alizarin-cleared preparation. Anterior part of the body, dorsal view. Newborn. *S* = suproccipitale, *B* = basioccipitale, *Ex* = exoccipitale, *D* = ossification center in basis of dens (*black point*).
KT 891

0.5 mm

In the *sternum* the sternebrae have enlarged considerably. When the ribs grow slightly asymmetrical, the sternebrae are correspondingly asymmetrical ("crankshaft-sternum," Fig. 308). In the *fore-* and *hindfeet*, nearly all bones of the phalanges have formed. The metacarpalia and metatarsalia had already appeared previously. Only the centers of the fifth middle phalanx (hindfeet) and of the first phalanx (forefeet) are absent.

The *carpals* have not yet ossified. In the *tarsus*, however, 2 ossification centers can be seen regularly: the talus and calcaneus. They are distinctively large, even though they have just recently appeared (Fig. 286).

Placenta

The structure of the placenta has not changed fundamentally since the 14-day stage (Fig. 309). Reichert's membrane usually ruptures shortly before birth. When it ruptures, it often rolls up like a carpet. Where it borders the placenta, however, the membrane remains stretched (Fig. 311). In the vicinity of the placental margin, short processes in Reichert's membrane appear at 14 days (Fig. 309).

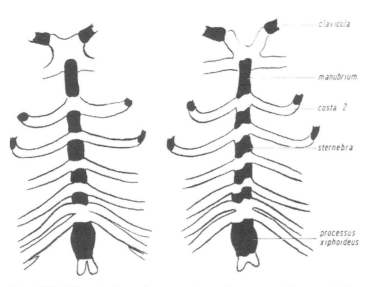

FIG. 308. Alizarin-cleared preparation of sternum. Note variable, but normal form of ossification centers ("crankshaft-sternum").
KT 865, 891

140

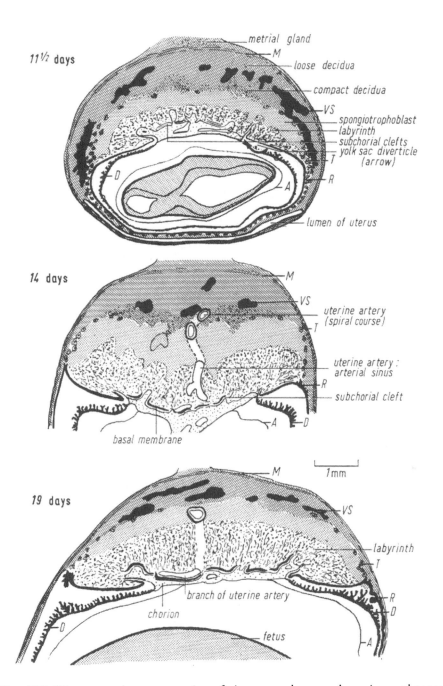

FIG. 309. Diagrammatic representation of placenta and extraembryonic membranes, from 11 1/2 days to birth.

M = muscle layer, *VS* = venous sinus, *T* = trophoblastic giant cells, *R* = Reichert's membrane, *D* = yolk sac, *A* = amnion.

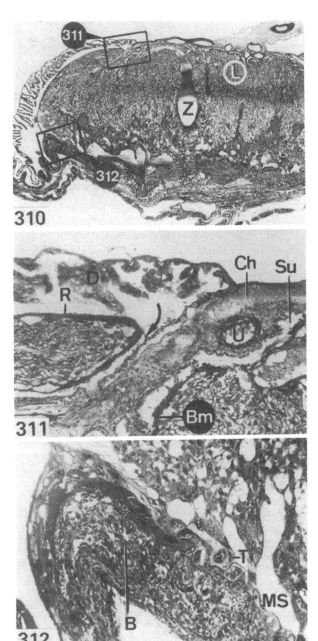

FIG. 310. Cross section through placenta of a newborn mouse, low power.
L = labyrinth, Z = central artery.
KT 1056. 14.5:1

FIG. 311. High power view of chorionic plate (*Ch*).
D = yolk sac, visceral layer; R = Reichert's membrane; *Bm* = basal membrane; U = umbilical vessel; *Su* = subchorionic space. *Arrow* indicates "yolk sac diverticle."
105:1

FIG. 312. High power view of basal plate (B).
MS = maternal blood sinus, T = trophoblastic giant cell. 105:1

At *19 days*, the placenta has not enlarged much. A dilated central artery enters the well-developed labyrinth from the mesometrial side of the placenta. This vessel conducts maternal blood directly under the chorionic plate, where the stems of the umbilical vessels pass. The labyrinth is demarcated from the chorionic plate by the narrow intraplacental space [33]. This space consists of subchorionic clefts bordered by two walls of characteristic structure. Toward the chorion, one wall is lined by a layer of cuboidal cells. Toward the labyrinth, the other wall is lined by flattened epithelial cells supported by a thick basement membrane (Fig. 311). The intraplacental space opens laterally into the lumen of the yolk sac [33], ("yolksac diverticles," marked by *arrow* in Fig. 311).

The *labyrinth* is composed of an intricate maternal blood space and numerous fetal blood vessels. Maternal and embryonic blood is separated by three cell layers, as shown by electron microscopic studies [34]. Two syncytial layers, which are closely approximated, are covered, near the maternal blood space, by single large trophoblastic cells.

The *spongiotrophoblast* (reticular zone or junctional zone) [38] contains exclusively maternal blood vessels. Large veins open from the decidua into extended (maternal) lacunae.

At the margins of the placenta, the spongiotrophoblast is bounded by the characteristic *giant cells* [39] mentioned above (Fig. 312).

142

Stage 28   Postnatal Development

Within 3 days, a fine fur appears and the *ears* are opening. The internal ear is still quite immature. The definitive histologic structure does not develop until 13 days. The *retina* is also immature.

The *eyes* open at 12 to 14 days.

At 6 weeks, the vagina opens, and females begin estrous cycles. The first successful mating takes place at 2 or 3 months of age.

The *skeleton* is used here as a convenient index of relative stages of postnatal development. Mice of 7 and 24 days were chosen arbitrarily to be described.

7 Days Post Partum

The linear length (head to base of the tail) is about 38 mm.

At 7 days the distal epiphyseal centers appear in the tibia and fibula (Fig. 315). In the tail, 24 *vertebrae* have ossification centers. Our adult hybrids have:

30–31 tail vertebrae

4 sacral vertebrae

6 lumbar vertebrae

13 thoracic vertebrae

7 cervical vertebrae

The neural arches of the sacral vertebrae are about to fuse, while the lumbar arches are still well separated (Fig. 314). The ossification centers of the vertebral bodies are separated throughout from the centers of the arches by narrow epiphyseal plates (Fig. 318). The discrete horizontal cleft separating the two centers of the axis (i.e., base of the body and base of the dens) is difficult to recognize (Fig. 314).

Extremities

Since birth, numerous ossification centers have appeared as seen in Figs. 315 and 317. The distal epiphyseal centers in the *tibia* and fibula are typical for 7-day mice. They appear shortly after the distal epiphyseal center of the femur.

In the tarsus, not only are the talus and calcaneus visible in alizarin-stained cleared preparations, but also the cuboid, 3 cuneiformia, and naviculare. The os tibiale, however, has not yet ossified.

In the *ovary*, there are abundant primary follicles in the cortical zone. In deeper areas, some (secondary) follicles are growing, but Graafian follicles are still lacking (Fig. 316).

There is little change in the *testis* since birth. Many cells have entered prophase. Spermiogenesis will start at 9 days of age.

In the *thymus* a few small Hassal's corpuscles can be seen (Fig. 319).

FIG. 313. 7-day old mouse female.
KT 893. 1.6:1

FIG. 314. Alizarin-cleared preparation, 7 days post partum, dorsal view.
S = supraoccipitale, Ax = 2 ossification centers of axis (axis body and basis of dens), At = processus transversus atlantis, U = ossification center in olecranon (ulna), L_2 = body of second lumbar vertebra, OJ = os ilii, Is = os ichii.
KT 893. 1.6:1

FIG. 315. Same skeleton as in Fig. 314, lateral view.
Fe = ossification center in distal epiphysis of femur; TF = ossification centers in distal epiphysis of tibia and fibula, having newly arisen; Ta = tarsalia (7 ossification centers, partially hidden). 1.6:1

FIG. 316. Ovary, showing secondary follicles, located near central region, 7 days post partum.
KT 892. 105:1

FIG. 317. Thorax, ventral view, 7 days post partum. Alizarin-cleared preparation.
Initial calcification of rib cartilage (R). Tm = apophyseal center in tuberculum maius, E = epiphyseal center in caput humeri, Co = ossification center in coracoid process (below clavicula), Ma = manubrium sterni, Xi = xiphoid process.
KT 893. 5:1

FIG. 318. Lumbar vertebrae, ventral view, Alizarin-cleared preparation, 7 days post partum.
L_2 = body of 2nd lumbar vertebra, Ar = arch-center of 2nd lumbar vertebra, OJ = os ilii, Is = os ischii, P = os pubis.
KT 893. 5:1

144

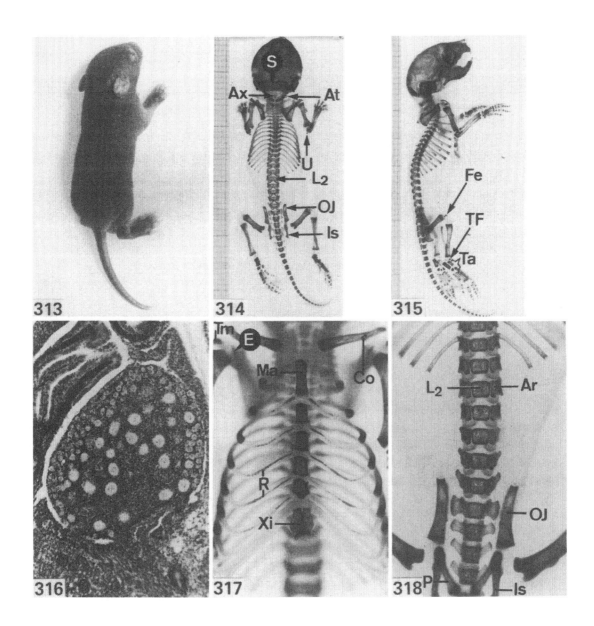

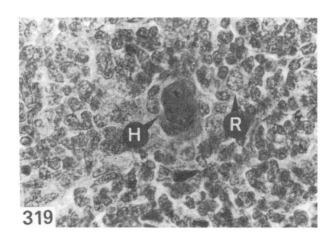

FIG. 319. Hassal's corpuscule (*H*) within thymus of 7-day-old mouse.
R = reticulum cell.
KT 892. 700:1

In the *eye*, the external plexiform layer is beginning to form, and it can be recognized for the first time. As a consequence, the nuclear zone becomes subdivided into external and internal nuclear zones. The process of separation starts centrally, near the optic nerve, and proceeds quickly towards the periphery. On the 11th day after birth, the outer segments of the photoreceptor cells are forming.

At 14 days, the rods have attained their final length.

In the internal *ear*, the organ of Corti is differentiating [180]. Differentiation starts at birth and is complete at 13 days (Figs. 324–326).

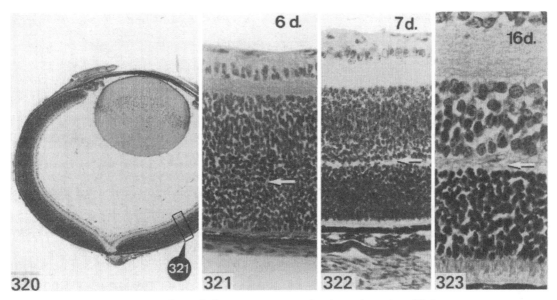

FIG. 320. Low power view of eye, 6 days post partum, horizontal section. 28:1

FIG. 321. High power view of retina of FIG. 320.
Arrows in Figs. 321–323 indicate development of outer plexiform layer, separating inner and outer nuclear layers. 240:1

FIG. 322. At 7 days, the nuclear layers are distinctly separated.
KT 892. 240:1

FIG. 323. Fully differentiated retina, 16 days post partum. 500:1

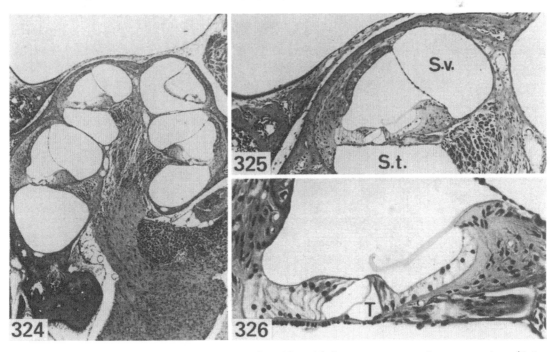

FIG. 324. Longitudinal section through axis of cochlea, 16 days post partum, low power view. 40:1

FIG. 325. High power view of cochlear duct (apical part) of FIG. 324.
S.v. = scala vestibuli, *S.t.* = scala tympani. 150:1

FIG. 326. High power view of organ of Corti of FIG. 325.
T = inner tunnel. 270:1

24 Days Post Partum

The linear length (head to base of tail) ranges from 50–60 mm.

At this age, the animals may be weaned.

The *vertebral column* continues to grow. In microscopic preparations, large cartilaginous growth zones are visible. The tail has attained its full number of 30 osseous vertebrae. There are only 4 pairs of hemal arch bones. These are small spherical pieces of bone bilaterally situated ventral to the caudal intervertebral discs. They develop first in the proximal part of the tail.

In the tarsus, the appearance of the apophysis of the tuber calcanei is a characteristic of this age (Fig. 329). In the lower and upper thigh of cleared animals, distinct epiphyseal plates can be seen. There are also epiphyseal plates in the acetabulum (Fig. 330).

Numerous blood vessels have grown into the flat epiphyses of the sacral and of the adjacent caudal vertebrae (Fig. 332).

In the *testes* there is active spermatogenesis. At 13 days after birth, differentiated *Sertoli cells* may be recognized. The original large and centrally placed primordial germ cells give rise to smaller, peripherally situated *spermatogonia*.

Many gonocytes have entered meiotic prophase. At the same time, the seminiferous tubules are developing lumina.

At 24 days there are no spermatozoa, but some tubules contain numerous young spermatids. Some peritubular cells are now transforming into smooth muscle cells (M.H. Ross [106]). In the *ovary*, primary, secondary (growing) and tertiary (Graafian) follicles can be recognized (Fig. 331). The oocytes are in dictyotene stage. Occasionally, multinucleate eggs may be seen. I have seen them only in follicles containing numerous pycnotic and degenerating granulosa cells. These follicles will probably soon degenerate. The growing follicle in Fig. 331 also shows signs of atresia.

FIG. 327. Hybrid female mouse, 24 days post partum.

FIG. 328. Alizarin-cleared preparation, lateral view, male, 24 days post partum. Right extremities removed, millimeter scale.
KT 899

FIG. 329. Dorsal view of skeleton, before removing right extremities.
Ap = apophyseal center in tuber calcanei.
KT 899. 1.5:1

FIG. 330. Ventral view of skeleton, enlarged, 24 days post partum.
M = manubrium sterni, *H* = acetabulum with epiphyseal plates.
KT 899. 2.7:1

FIG. 331. Section through ovary, 24 days post partum. Hematoxylin-Eosin.
T = tertiary follicle (Graafian follicle), *P* = polynucleate oocyte, in secondary follicle.
KT 1071. 105:1

FIG. 332. Intervertebral disc of proximal tail. Frontal section at 4 weeks.
CH = notochordal sheath within epiphyseal plate of 2nd caudal vertebra, *G* = blood vessels in epiphyseal plate of first caudal vertebra.
KT 787a. 105:1

148

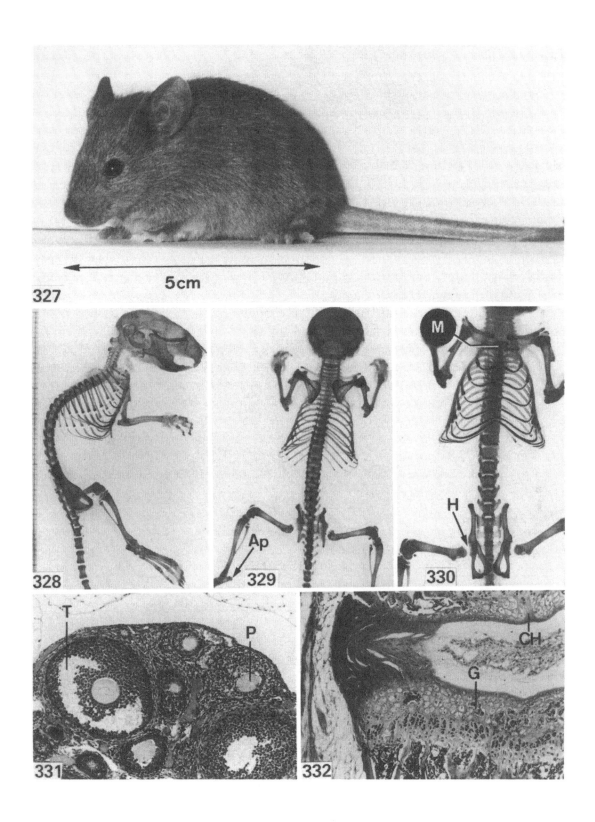

327

328

329
Ap

330
M
H

331
T
P

332
CH
G

29 Weight Curves

The mouse has reached its full size at 3–4 months. The growth curve is dependent on genetic (Fig. 333) and environmental [3] factors, especially the amount of milk available [198]. The temperature also has some influence on growth [201].

The males become heavier than the females at the age of 4 weeks.

Specific pathogen-free (SPF) animals seem to grow faster than conventionally reared mice. Before we established our SPF colony, our CBAs had a considerably lower growth rate than the C57BL/6J animals. Now, in pathogen-free colonies, the CBAs grow faster than the C57BL/6J mice. Environmental factors may play an unexpected role in the growth rate of mice. They are difficult to take into account in applying a mathematical model [196] to the growth of inbred mice (Fig. 334).

Pregnant females begin to gain appreciable weight from the 8th day of pregnancy (Fig. 335). Like growth rate, *life span* is influenced by many genetic and environmental factors. It may vary between 1 and 3 years [2].

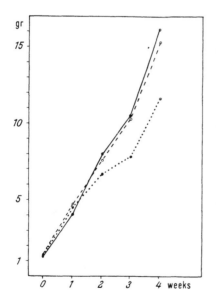 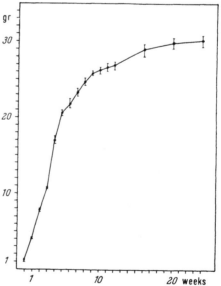

FIG. 333. Mean weights of our growing inbred and hybrid mice. Hybrids (*full line*) show maximum increase in weight. *Broken line* indicates CBA; *stippled line* indicates C57BL/6.

FIG. 334. Postnatal increase in weight of our hybrid males.
Short perpendicular lines indicate standard errors.

150

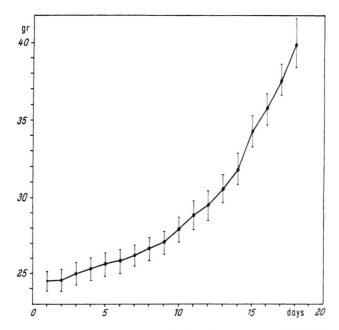

FIG. 335. Increase in weight of pregnant hybrids (C57BL/6-females). *Short perpendicular lines* indicate standard errors.

Selected References

Opera Generalia

1. Cook, M.J.: The anatomy of the laboratory mouse, 143 p. London–New York: Academic Press 1965.
2. Green, E.L.: Biology of the laboratory mouse, 706 p. New York: McGraw Hill 1966.
3. Gruneberg, H.: The genetics of the mouse, 2nd ed., 650 p. The Hague: Martinus Nijhoff 1952.
4. Otis, E.M., Brent, R.: Equivalent ages in mouse and human embryos. Anat. Rec. 120, 33–64 (1952).
5. Rugh, R.: The mouse. Its reproduction and development, 430 p. Minneapolis: Burgess 1968.
6. Streeter, G.L.: Developmental horizons in human embryos. Contr. Embryol. Carneg. Instn. 30, 213–230 (1942)

Preimplantation Period

7. Austin, C.R.: Fertilization, 145 p. Englewood, N.Y.: Prentice-Hall 1965.
8. Beatty, R.A., Sharma, K.N.: Genetic of gametes. III. Stain differences in spermatozoa from eight inbred strains of mice. Proc. roy. Soc. Edinb. B 68, 27–53 (1960).
9. Beatty, R.A., Fischberg, M.: Heteroploidy in mammals. III. Induction of tetraploidy in pre-implantation mouse eggs. J. Genet. 50, 471–479 (1952).
10. Calarco, P.G., Brown, E.H.: An ultrastructural and cytological study of pre-implantation development of the mouse. J. exp. Zool. 171, 253–284 (1969).
11. Chang, M.C., Hunt, D.M.: Morphological changes of sperm head in the ooplasm of mouse, rat, hamster and rabbit. Anat. Rec. 142, 417–426 (1962).
12. Dickson, A.D.: The form of the mouse blastocyst. J. Anat. (Lond.) 100, 335–348 (1966).
13. Dickson, A.D.: Variation in development of mouse blastocysts. J. Anat. (Lond.) 101, 263–267 (1967).
14. Edwards, R.G.: Timing of stages of maturation division, ovulations, fertilization and the first cleavage of eggs of adult mice treated with gonadotropins, J. Endocr. 18, 272–304 (1959).
15. Graham, C.F.: Parthenogenetic mouse blastocysts. Nature (Lond.) 226, 165–167 (1970).
16. Lewis, W.H., Wright, E.S.: On the early development of the mouse egg. Contr. Embryol. Carneg. Instn. 25, 113–143 (1935).
17. Potts, D.M., Wilson, J.B.: The pre-implantation conceptus of the mouse at 90 hours post coitum. J. Anat. (Lond.) 102, 1–11 (1967).
18. Stevens, L.C.: The development of teratomas from intra-testicular grafts of 2-cell mouse eggs. Anat. Rec. 157, 328 (abstr.) (1967).
19. Weitlauf, H.M.: Temporal changes in protein synthesis by mouse blastocysts transferred to ovariectomized recipients. J. exp. Zool. 171, 481–486 (1969).
20. Whitten, W.K., Biggers, J.D.: Complete development in vitro of the pre-implantation stages of the mouse in a simple chemically defined medium. J. Reprod. Fertil. 17, 399–401 (1958).
21. Wolstenholme, G.E.W., O'Connor, M.: Pre-implantation stages of pregnancy. Ciba Foundation Symposium, 430 p. London: J. & A. Churchill Ltd. 1965.

Implantation and Fetal Membranes

22. Amoroso, E.C.: Placentation. In: A.S. Parkes (edit.), Marshall's physiology of reproduction, 3rd edit., vol. 2, p. 127–311. London: Longmans, Green 1952.
23. Arvis, G.: Les cellules ultratrophoblastiques. Etude ultrastructurale au cours de la nidation chez la souris. C.R. Ass. Anat. 55e Congr. No 147, 87–104 (1970).
24. Billlingham, W.D., Kirby, D.R.S., Owen, J.J.T., Ritter, M.A., Burtonshaw, M.D., Evans, E.P., Ford, C.E., Gauld, I.K., McLaren, A.: Placental barrier to maternal cells. Nature (Lond.) 244, 704–706 (1969).
25. Bloch, S.: Die Glandula myometralis im Uterus der Maus. Acta anat. (Basel) 56, 103–119 (1964).
26. Bloch, S.: Beobachtungen zur Wechselwirkung zwischen Keim und Uterus bei der Implantation. Acta anat. (Basel) 65, 594–605 (1966).
27. Boyd, J.D., Hamilton, W.J.: Cleavage, early development and implantation of the egg. In: A.S. Parkes (edit.), Marshall's physiology of reproduction, 3rd edit., vol. 2, p. 1–126. London: Longmans, Green 1952.
28. Calarco, P., Moyer, F.H.: Structural changes in the murine yolk sac during gestation: Cytochemical and electron microscope observations. J. Morph. 119, 341–356 (1966).
29. Chiquoine, A.D.: The distribution of polysaccharides during gastrulation and embryogenesis in the mouse embryo. Anat. Rec. 129, 495–516 (1957).
30. Dean, H.W., RRubin, B.L., Dirks, E.C., Lober, B.L., Leipner, G.: Trophoblastic giant cells in placentas of rat and mice and their probable role in steroid hormone production. Endocrinology 70, 407–419 (1962).
31. Enders, A.C.: A comparative study of the fine structure of the trophoblast in several hemochorial placentas. Amer. J. Anat. 116, 29–68 (1965).
32. Finn, C.A., McLaren, A.: A study of early stages of implantation in mice. J. Reprod. Fertil. 13, 259–267 (1967).
33. Friedrich, F.: Die Entwicklung der sogenannten Dottersackdivertikel in der Plazenta der weißen Maus. Z. Anat. Entwickl.-Gesch. 124, 153–170 (1964).
34. Kirby, D., Bradbury, S.: The hemochorial mouse placenta. Anat. Rec. 152, 279–282 (1965).
35. Porter, D.G.: Observations on the development of mouse blastocysts transferred to the testis and kidney. Amer. J. Anat. 121, 73–86 (1967).
36. Reinius, S.: Morphology of the mouse embryo, from the time of implantation to mesoderm formation. Z. Zellforsch. 68, 711–723 (1965).
37. Reinius, S.: Ultrastructure of blastocyst attachment in the mouse. Z. Zellforsch. 77, 257–266 (1967).
38. Saccoman, F., Morgan, C.F., Wells, L.J.: Radioautographic studies of DNA-Synthesis in the developing extra-embryonic membranes of the mouse. Anat. Rec. 158, 197–206 (1967).
39. Schiebler, H.: Mitteilungen über die Riesenzellen der Nagetierplazenta. Verh. Anat. Ges. 54. Verslg. Anat. Anz., Erg.-H. 104, 318–323 (1958).
40. Smith, L.J.: Metrial gland and other glycogen containing cells in the mouse uterus following mating, and through implantation of the embryo. Amer. J. Anat. 119, 15–23 (1966).
41. Theiler, K.: Die Anlage des Vorderdarmes bei der Hausmaus, und die Furchenbildungen am Eizylinder. Z. Anat. Entwickl.-Gesch. 128, 40–46 (1969).

Blood and Circulatory System

42. Albert, S., Wolf, P.L., Potter, R.: Observations on the origin of lymphocyte-like cells in the mouse bone marrow. Nature (Lond.) 212, 1577–1579 (1966).
43. Andrews, W.: Comparative hematology. New York: Grune & Stratton 1965.
44. Bermann, J.: The ultrastructure of erythroblastic islands and reticular cells in mouse bone marrow. J. Ultrastruct. Res. 17, 291–313 (1967).

45. Caruso, R., Petrakis, N.L.: Studies of the coagulation and prothrombin time in the mouse embryo. Thrombos. Diathes. haemorrh. (Stuttg.) 16, 732–737 (1966).
46. Chapelle, A. de la, Fantoni, A., Marks, P.A.: Differentiation of mammalian somatic cells: DNA and hemoglobin synthesis in fetal mouse yolk sac erythroid cells. Proc. nat. Acad. Sci. (Wash.) 63, 812–819 (1969).
47. Craig, M.L.: A developmental change in hemoglobins, correlated with an embryonic red cell population in the mouse. Develop. Biol. 10, 191–201 (1964).
48. Orlic, D., Gordon, A.S., Rhodin, J.A.G.: An ultrastructural study of erythropoietin-induced red cell formation in mouse spleen. J. Ultrastruct. Res. 13, 516–542 (1965).
49. Ravn, E.: Über die Arteria omphalo-mesenterica der Ratten und Mäuse. Anat. Anz. 9, 420–429 (1894).
50. Salzer, P., Theiler, K.: Über eine besondere Klappe am Ductus venosus Arantii bei der Maus. Z. Anat. Entwickl.-Gesch. 130, 91–94 (1970).

Lymph Nodes, Thymus, Spleen

51. Burnet, F.M.: Mast cells in the mouse thymus. In: G.E.W. Wolstenholme and R. Porter, The thymus, p. 335–340. Boston: Little & Brown 1966.
52. Crisan, C.: Die Entwicklung des thyreo-parathyreothymischen Systems der weißen. Maus. Z. Anat. Entwickl.-Gesch. 104, 327–358 (1935).
53. Dunn, T.B.: Normal and pathologic anatomy of the reticular tissue in laboratory mice with a classification and discussion of neoplasms. J. nat. Cancer Inst. 14, 1281–1434 (1954).
54. Engeset, H., Tjotta, E.: Lymphatic pathways from the tail in rats and mice. Cancer Res. 20, 613–614 (1960).
55. Mandel, T.: Differentiation of epithelial cells in the mouse thymus. Z. Zellforsch. 106, 498–517 (1970).
56. Miyazaki, T.: Über die Entwicklung der Lymphknoten bei der Maus. Soc. Path. Jap. Trans. 30, 29–34 (1940).
57. Prindull, G.: Die Milz als nachgeordnetes lymphatisches Organ. Z. Anat. Entwickl.-Gesch. 125, 255–275 (1966).
58. Sanel, F.T.: Ultrastructure of differentiating cells during thymus histogenesis. Z. Zellforsch. 83, 8–29 (1967).
59. Sanel, F.T., Copenhaver, W.M.: Histogenesis of mouse thymus studied with the light and electron microscope. Anat. Rec. 151, 410 (abstr.) (1965).
60. Smith, C.: Studies on the thymus of the mammals. XIV. Histology and histochemistry of embryonic and early postnatal thymus of C57BL/6 and AKR strain mice. Amer. J. Anat. 116, 611–629 (1965).

Palate and Respiratory Tract

61. Browder, S.: Factors influencing lung lobation in the mouse. I. Genetic factors. A preliminary report. Anat. Rec. 83, 31–39 (1942).
62. Callas, G., Walker, B.E.: Palate morphogenesis in mouse embryos after irradiation. Anat. Rec. 145, 61–68 (1963).
63. Crocker, T.T., Teeter, A., Nielsen, B.: Postnatal cellular proliferation in mouse and hamster lung. Cancer Res. 30, 357–361 (1970).
64. Farbman, A.J.: The epithelium-connective tissue interface during closure of the secondary palate in rodent embryos. J. dent. Res. 48, 617–624 (1969).
65. Jacobs, R.M.: Histochemical study of morphogenesis and teratogenesis of the palate in mouse embryos. Anat. Rec. 149, 691–698 (1964).
66. Karrer, H.E.: The ultrastructure of mouse lung: The alveolar macrophage. J. biophys. biochem. Cytol. 4, 693–700 (1958).

67. Larson, K.S.: Studies on the closure of the secondary palate. Exp. Cell Res. 21, 498–503 (1960).
68. Roos, L.M., Walker, B.E.: Movement of palatine shelves in untreated and teratogen-treated mouse embryos. Amer. J. Anat. 121, 509–522 (1967).
69. Trasler, D.G.: Pathogenesis of cleft lip and its relation to embryonic face shape in A/J and C57BL mice. Teratology 1, 33–50 (1968).
70. Walker, B.E.: Correlation of embryonic movement with palate closure in mice. Teratology 2, 191–198 (1968).

Teeth, Oral Cavity

71. Bader, R.S.: Fluctuating asymmetry in the dentition of the house mouse. Growth 29, 291–300 (1965).
72. Caramia, F.: Ultrastructure of mouse submaxillary gland. I. Sexual differences. J. Ultrastruct. Res. 16, 505–523 (1966).
73. Cohn, S.A.: Development of the molar teeth in the albino mouse. Amer. J. Anat. 101, 295–320 (1957).
74. Disher, L.: Histogenesis of the mouse submandibular salivary gland. Anat. Rec. 157, 235 (abstr.) (1967).
75. Gaunt, W.A.: The disposition of the developing cheek teeth in the albino mouse. Acta anat. (Basel) 64, 572–585 (1966).
76. Hinrichsen, K.: Morphologische Untersuchungen zur Topogenese der mandibularen Nagezähne der Maus. Anat. Anz. 107, 55–74 (1959).
77. Kelemen, G.: Nonexperimental nasal and paranasal pathology in hereditarily obese mice. Acta oto-laryng. (Stockh.) 57, 143–151 (1953).
78. Kutuzow, H., Sicher, H.: Comparative anatomy of the mucosa of the tongue and the palate of the laboratory mouse. Anat. Rec. 116, 409–425 (1953).
79. Weber, J., Kittel, R.: Die Abhängigkeit des Sekretionszyklus der Streifenstücke in der Glandula submandibularis vom ovariellen Zyklus der weißen Maus. Morph. Jb. 108, 1–17 (1965).

Intestinal Tract

80. Daems, W.T., Wisse, E.: Shape and attachment of the cristae mitochondriales in mouse hepatic cell mitochondria. J. Ultrastruct. Res. 16, 123–140 (1966).
81. Danforth, C.H., Center, E.: Development and genetics of a sexinfluenced trait in the livers of mice. Proc. nat. Acad. Sci. (Wash.) 39, 811–817 (1953).
82. Frankenberger, Z.: Sur la morphologie et le développement des voies biliaires chez le genre Mus. Arch. Anat. (Strasbourg) 6, 201–216 (1926).
83. Green, M.: A defect of the splanchnic mesoderm caused by the mutant gene dominant hemimelia in the mouse. Develop. Biol. 15, 62–89 (1966).
84. Moog, F.: The functional differentiation of the small intestine. II. The differentiation of alkaline phospho-monoesterase in the duodenum of the mouse. J. exp. Zool. 118, 187–207 (1951).
85. Overton, J.: Fine structure of the free cell surface in developing mouse intestinal mucosa. J. exp. Zool. 159, 195–202 (1965).
86. Parakkal, P.F.: An electron microscopic study of esophageal epithelium in the newborn and adult mouse. Amer. J. Anat. 121, 175–196 (1967).
87. Rutter, W.J., Wessells, N.K., Grobstein, C.: Control of specific synthesis in the developing pancreas. Nat. Cancer Inst. Monogr. 13, 51–65 (1964).
88. Theiler, K.: Die Anlage des Vorderdarmes bei der Hausmaus und die Furchenbildungen am Eizylinder. Z. Anat. Entwickl.-Gesch. 128, 40–46 (1969).
89. Wilson, J.W.: Abnormal mitosis in mouse liver. Amer. J. Anat. 86, 51–74 (1950).
90. Yamada, E.: The fine structure of the gall bladder epithelium of the mouse. J. biophys. biochem. Cytol. 1, 445–458 (1955).

Urogenital Tract

91. Brown, A.L.: An analysis of the developing metanephros in mouse embryos with abnormal kidneys. Amer. J. Anat. 47, 117–172 (1931).
92. Crabtree, C.: The structure of Bowman's capsule as an index of age and sex variations in normal mice. Anat. Rec. 79, 395–413 (1941).
93. Deane, H.W., Wurzelmann, S.: Electron microscopic observations on the postnatal differentiation of the seminal vesicle epithelium of the laboratory mouse. Amer. J. Anat. 117, 91–134 (1965).
94. Dunn, T.B.: Some observations of the normal and pathologic anatomy of the kidney of the mouse. J. nat. Cancer Inst. 9, 285–301 (1949).
95. Espinasse, P.G.: The oviduct epithelium of the mouse. J. Anat. (Lond.) 69, 363–368 (1935).
96. Firlitt, C.F., Davis, J.R.: Morphogenesis of the residual body of the mouse testis. Quart. J. micr. Sci. 106, 93–98 (1965).
97. Flickinger, C.J.: The postnatal development of the Sertoli cells of the mouse. Z. Zellforsch. 78, 92–113 (1967).
98. Forsberg, J.G., Olivecrona, H.: Further studies on the differentiation of the epithelium in the mouse vaginal anlage. Z. Zellforsch. 66, 867–877 (1965).
99. Fuxe, K., Nilsson, O.: The mouse uterine surface epithelium during the estrous cycle. Anat. Rec. 145, 541–548 (1963).
100. Grobstein, C.: Inductive interaction in the development of the mouse metanephros. J. exp. Zool. 130, 319–339 (1955).
101. Heinecke, H., Grimm, H.: Untersuchungen zur Öffnungszeit der Vaginalmembran bei verschiedenen Mäusestämmen. Endocrinology 35, 205–213 (1958).
102. Ludwig, E.: Beitrag zur Entwicklulngsgeschichte der Nachniere. Acta ana. (Basal) 8, 1–17 (1949).
103. Mintz, B.: Germ cell origin and history in the mouse: genetic and histochemical evidence. Anat. Rec. 127, 335–336 (abstr.) (1957).
104. Pierce, G.B., Beals, T.F.: The ultrastructure of primordial germinal cells of the fetal testes and of embryonal carcinoma cells of mice. Cancer Res. 24, 1553–1567 (1964).
105. Raynaud, A.: Développement des glandes annexes du tractus génital de la souris. C.R. Soc. Biol. (Basel) 136, 292–294 (1942).
106. Ross, M.H.: The fine structure and development of the peritubular contractile cell component in the seminiferous tubules of the mouse. Amer. J. Anat. 121, 523–558 (1967).
107. Wimsatt, W.A., Waldo, C.M.: The normal occurrence of a peritoneal opening in the bursa ovarii of the mouse. Anat. Rec. 93, 47–57 (1945).

Spermatogenesis

108. Cutright, P.R.: Spermatogenesis in the mouse. J. Morph. 54, 197–220 (1952).
109. Evans, E.P., Breckon, G., Ford, C.E.: An air-drying method for meiotic preparations from mammalian testes. Cytogenetics 3, 289–294 (1964).
110. Fogg, L.C., Cowing, R.F.: Cytological changes in the spermatogonial nuclei correlated with increased radioresistance. Exp. Cell Res. 4, 107–115 (1952).
111. Galton, M., Holt, S.F.: Asynchronous replication of the mouse sex chromosomes. Exp. Cell Res. 37, 111–116 (1965).
112. Gardner, P.J.: Fine structure of the seminiferous tubule of the Swiss mouse. The spermatid. Anat. Rec. 155, 235–250 (1966).
113. Lam, D.M.K., Furrer, R., Bruce, W.R.: The separation, physical characterization and differentiation kinetics of spermatogonial cells of the mouse. Proc. nat. Acad. Sci. (Wash.) 65, 192–199 (1970).

114. Leblond, C.P., Clermont, G.C.: Spermiogenesis of rat, mouse, hamster and guinea-pig as revealed by the PAS-technique. Amer. J. Anat. 90, 167–216 (1952).

115. Monesi, V.: Autoradiographic study of DNA-synthesis and the cell cycle in spermatogonia and spermatocytes of mouse testis using Thymidin H₃. J. Cell Biol. 14, 1–18 (1962).

116. Oakberg, E.F.: A description of spermiogenesis in the mouse and its use in analysis of the cycle of the seminiferous epithelium and germ cell renewal. Amer. J. Anat. 99, 391–414 (1956).

117. Oakberg, E.F.: Duration of spermatogenesis in the mouse and timing of stages in the cycle of the seminiferous epithelium. Amer. J. Anat. 99, 507–516 (1956).

118. Sapsford, C.S.: Changes in the cells of the sex cords and seminiferous tubules during the development of the testis of the rat and the mouse. Austral. J. Zool. 10, 178–192 (1962).

119. Sawada, T.: An electron microscope study of spermatid differentiation in the mouse. Okajimas Folia anat. jap. 30, 73–80 (1957).

120. Slizynski, B.M.: A preliminary pachytene chromosome map of the house mouse. J. Genet. 49, 242–244 (1949).

121. Sugihara, R., Yasuzumi, G.: The fine structure of nuclei as revealed by electron microscopy. VI. Relationship between nucleolus formation and sex chromosomes in the type "A" mouse spermatogonia. Z. Zellforsch. 107, 466–478 (1970).

Oogenesis

122. Ben-Or, S.: Morphological and functional development of the ovary of the mouse. J. Embryol. exp. Morph. 11, 715–740 (1963).

123. Borum, K.: Oogenesis in the mouse; a study of the origin of the mature ova. Exp. Cell Res. 45, 39–47 (1967).

124. Kent, H.A., Jr.: Polyovular follicles and multinucleate ova in the ovaries of young mice. Anat. Rec. 137, 521–524 (1960).

125. McLaren, A.: The distribution of eggs and embryos between sides in the mouse. J. Endocr. 27, 157–181 (1963).

126. Odor, D.L., Blandau, R.J.: Ultrastructural studies on fetal and early postnatal mouse ovaries. Amer. J. Anat. 125, 177–216 (1969).

Endocrine Glands

127. Carvalheira, A.F., Pearse, A.G.E.: Calcitonin. Symposium on thyreocalcitonin acid C-cells (S. Taylor, ed.), p. 122–126. London: W. Heinemann 1967.

128. Chardard-Ramboult, S.: Développement de la glande thyroïde chez la souris pendant la vie intra-utérine. C.R. Soc. Biol. (Paris) 143, 40–41 (1949).

129. Coupland, R.E.: The post-natal distribution of the abdominal chromaffine tissue in the guinea-pig, mouse and white rat. J. Anat. (Lond.) 94, 244–256 (1960).

130. Delost, P., Chirvan-Nia, P.: Différences raciales dans l'involution de la zone X surrénalienne chez la souris adulte vièrge. C.R. Soc. Biol. (Paris) 152, 453–455 (1958).

131. Dunn, T.B.: Ciliated cells of the thyroid of the mouse. J. nat. Cancer Inst. 4, 555–557 (1944).

132. Ekholm, R.: The ultrastructure of the blood capillaries in the mouse thyroid gland. Z. Zellforsch. 46, 139–146 (1957).

133. Gorbman, A.: Functional and morphological properties in the thyroid gland, ultimobranchial body, and persisting ductus pharyngo-branchialis IV. of adult mouse. Anat. Rec. 98, 93–101 (1947).

134. Hitzemann, S.J.W.: Development of enzyme activity in the Leydig cells of mouse testis. Anat. Rec. 143, 351–361 (1962).

135. Jacobs, B.B.: Variations in thyroid morphology of mice. Proc. Soc. exp. Biol. (N.Y.) 97, 115–118 (1958).

136. Kerr, T.: The development of the pituitary of the laboratory mouse. Quart. J. micr. Sci. 87, 3–29 (1946).
137. McPhail, M.K., Read, H.G.: The mouse adrenal. I. Development, degeneration and regeneration of the X-zone. Anat. Rec. 84, 51–73 (1942).
138. Mirskaia, L., Crew, F.A.E.: Maturity in the female mouse. Proc. Roy. Soc. (Edinb.) 50, 179–186 (1930).
139. Munger, B.L.: A light and electron microscopic study of cellular differentiation in the pancreatic islets of the mouse. Amer. J. Anat. 103, 275–312 (1958).
140. Ross, M.H.: Fine structure of the juxta-medullary region of the mouse adrenal cortex with special reference to the X-zone. Anat. Rec. 157, 313 (abstract) (1967).
141. Sano, M., Sasaki, F.: Embryonic development of the mouse anterior pituitary studied by light and electron microscopy. Z. Anat. Entwickl.-Gesch. 129, 195–222 (1969).
142. Sato, T., Jshikawa, K., Aoi, T., Kitoh, J., Sugiyama, S.: Electron microscopic observations on the development of the parafollicular cells from the ultimobranchial cyst in the thyroid gland of the mouse. Okajimas Folia anat. jap. 42, 91–105 (1966).
143. Smith, C., Clifford, C.P.: Histochemical study of aberrant thyroid glands associated with the thymus of the mouse. Anat. Rec. 143, 229–238 (1962).
144. Smithberg, M., Brunner, M.N.: The induction and maintenance of pregnancy in prepuberal mice. J. exp. Zool. 133, 441–457 (1956).
145. Stoeckel, M.E., Porte, A.: Observations ultrastructurales sur la parathyroide de souris. I. Etude chez la souris normale. Z. Zellforsch. 73, 488–502 (1966).
146. Treilhou-Lahille, F., Zylberberg-Jeanmaire, R.: Histologie topographique des dérivés pharyngiens de 'lembryon de souris C57/BL entre le 12e et le 15e jour de gestation. C.R. Ass. Anat. 53e Congr., No 144, 1828–1834 (1969).
147. Van Heyningen, H.E.: The initiation of thyroid function in the mouse. Endocrinology 69, 720–727 (1961).
148. Von Bartheld, F., Moll, J.: The vascular system of the mouse epiphysis with remarks on the comparative anatomy of the venous trunks in the epiphyseal area. Acta anat. (Basel) 22, 227–235 (1954).
149. Waring, H.: The development of the adrenal gland of the mouse. Quart. J. micr. Sci. 78, 329–366 (1935).

Brain, Sensory Organs, Skin

150. Wessells, N.K., Roessner, K.D.: Non-proliferation in dermal condensations of mouse vibrissae and pelage hairs. Develop. Biol. 12, 419–433 (1965).
151. Billingham, R.E., Silvers, W.K.: The melanocytes of mammals. Quart. Rev. Biol. 35, 1–40 (1960).
152. Chase, H.B.: The behaviour of pigment cells and epithelial cells in the hair follicle. In: The biology of hair growth (chap. I). New York: Academic Press 1958.
153. Chase, H.B., Mann, S.J.: Phenogenetic aspects of some hair and pigment mutants. J. cell comp. Physiol. 56, 103–111 (1960).
154. Chiquoine, A.D.: Distribution of alkaline phosphomono-esterase in the central nervous system of the mouse embryo. J. comp. Neurol. 100, 415–440 (1954).
155. Cohen, A.J.: Electron microscopic observations of the developing mouse eye. I. Basement membranes during early development and lens formation. Develop. Biol. 3, 297–316 (1961).
156. De Long, B.R., Sidman, R.L.: Effects of eye removal at birth on histogenesis of the mouse superior colliculus: An autoradiographic analysis with tritiated Thymidine. J. comp. Neurol. 118, 205–224 (1962).
157. Fawcett, D.W.: A comparison of the histological organization and cytochemical reactions of brown and white adipose tissue. J. Morph. 90, 363–406 (1952).

158. Graumann, W.: Zelldegeneration im Telencephalon medium und Paraphysenentwicklung bei der weißen Maus. Z. Anat. Entwickl.-Gesch. 115, 19–31 (1950).

159. Hanna, C.: Changes in DNA, RNA and protein synthesis in the developing lens. Invest. Ophthal. 4, 480–495 (1965).

160. Herrlinger, H.: Licht- und elektronenmikroskopische Untersuchungen am Subcommissural-organ der Maus. Ergebn. Anat. Entwickl.-Gesch. 42, H. 5 (1970).

161. Kallen, B.: Notes on the development of the neural crest in the head of Mus musculus. J. Embryol. exp. Morph. 1, 393–398 (1953).

162. Kallen, B., Lindskog, B.: Formation and disappearance of neuromery in Mus musculus. Acta anat. (Basel) 18, 273–282 (1953).

163. Kaneko, K.: Über die Entwicklung der Thalamuskerne der Maus. Folia anat. jap. 19, 557–596 (1940).

164. Kovac, W., Denk, H.: Der Hirnstamm der Maus. Wien-New York: Springer 1968.

165. Knudsen, P.A.: Mode of growth of the choroid plexus in mouse embryos. Acta anat. (Basel) 57, 172–182 (1964).

166. Mattanza, G.: Über die Bedeutung des embryonalen Zellunterganges im Vorderhirn. Acta anat. (Basel) 85, 96–104 (1973).

167. Marsden, H.M., Silvers, W.K.: The effects of genotype and cell environment on melanoblast differentiation in the house mouse. Genetics 41, 429–450 (1956).

168. Melaragno, H.P., Montagna, W.: The tactile hair follicles in the mouse. Anat. Rec. 115, 129–150 (1953).

169. Meller, K., Breipohl, W., Glees, P.: Ontogeny of the mouse motor cortex. The polymorph layer or layer VI. A Golgi and electron-microscopic study. Z. Zellforsch. 99, 443–458 (1969).

170. Menefee, M.G.: The differentiation of keratin-containing cells in the epidermis of embryo mice. Anat. Rec. 122, 181–191 (1953).

171. Moyer, F.H.: Electron microscope studies on the origin, development and genetic control of melanin granules in the mouse eye. In: G.K. Smelser, The structure of the eye. New York: Academic Press 1961.

172. Niimi, K., Harada, I., Kusaka, Y., Kishi, S.: The ontogenetic development of the diencephalon in the mouse. Tokushima J. exp. Med. 8, 203–238 (1961).

173. Pierce, E.T.: Histogenesis of the nuclei grisei pontis, corporis pontobulbaris and reticularis tegmenti pontis (Bechterew) in the mouse. J. comp. Neurol. 126, 219–240 (1966).

174. Rawles, M.E.: Origin of pigment cells from the neural crest in the mouse. Physiol. Zool. 20, 248–266 (1947).

175. Richardson, F.L.: The acinar pattern in the mammary glands of virgin mice at different ages. J. nat. Cancer Inst. 38, 305–315 (1967).

176. Seifert, K., Ule, G.: Die Ultrastruktur der Riechschleimhaut der neugeborenen und jugendlichen weißen Maus. Z. Zellforsch. 76, 147–169 (1967).

177. Sidman, R.L.: Histogenesis of mouse retina. Studies with Thymidine-H3. In: The structure of the eye (G. Smelser). New York: Academic Press 1961.

178. Turner, C.W., Gomez, E.T.: The normal development of the mammary gland of the male and female albino mouse. Univ. Miss. Res. Bull. 182 (1932).

179. Uzmann, L.: The histogenesis of the mouse cerebellum as studied by its tritiated thymidine uptake. J. comp. Neurol. 114, 137–159 (1960).

180. Weibel, E.R.: Zur Kenntnis der Differenzierungsvorgänge im Epithel des Ductus cochlearis. Acta anat. (Basel) 29, 53–90 (1957).

181. Wrenn, J.T., Wessells, N.K.: An ultrastructural study of lens invagination in the mouse. J. exp. Zool. 171, 359–368 (1969).

Skeletal System, Musculature

182. Bateman, N.: Bone growth: A study of the grey-lethal and microphthalmic mutants in the mouse. J. Anat. (Lond.) 88, 212–260 (1954).

183. Chen, J.M.: Studies on the morphogenesis of the mouse sternum. I. Normal embryonic development. J. Anat. (Lond.) 86, 373–386 (1952).

184. Forsthoefel, P.F.: Observations on the sequence of blastemal condensations in the limbs of the mouse embryo. Anat. rec. 147, 129–138 (1963).

185. Frommer, J.: Prenatal development of the mandibular joint in mice. Anat. Rec. 150, 449–461 (1964).

186. Gruneberg, H.: The pathology of development. A study of inherited skeletal disorders in animals, 390 p. Oxford: Blackwell 1963.

187. Hoshino, K.: Comparative study on the skeletal development in the fetus of rat and mouse. Congenit Anomalies (Japan) 7, 32–38 (1967).

188. Johnson, M.L.: The time and order of appearance of ossification centers in the albino mouse. Amer. J. Anat. 52, 241–271 (1933).

189. Theiler, K.: Zelluntergang in den hintersten Rumpfsomiten bei der Maus. Z. Anat. Entwickl.-Gesch. 120, 274–278 (1958).

190. Theiler, K.: Experimentelle Segmentierungsstörungen. Verh. Anat. Ges. (Marburg 1967). Erg.-H. Anat. Anz. 121, 557–560 (1968).

191. Wirsen, C., Larsson, K.S.: Histochemical differentiation of skeletal muscle in foetal and newborn mice. J. Embryol. exp. Morph. 12, 759–767 (1964).

192. Wirtschafter, Z.T.: Genesis of the mouse skeleton. Springfield: Ch. C. Thomas 1966.

Growth

193. Atlas, M., Bond, V.P.: The cell generation cycle of the eleven-day mouse embryo. J. Cell Biol 26, 19–24 (1965).

194. Goedbloed, J.F.: La croissance de l'embryon du rat et de la souris, et quelques-uns de leurs organes, et la croissance post-natale de la souris. C.R. Ass. Anat. 53e Congr., No 142, 933–941 (1969).

195. Gruneberg, H.: A ventral ectodermal ridge of the tail in mouse embryos. Nature (Lond.) 177, 787–788 (1956).

196. Laird, A.K., Howard, A.: Growth curves in inbred mice. Nature (Lond.) 213, 786–788 (1967).

197. McDowell, E.C., Allen, E., McDowell, C.G.: The prenatal growth of the mouse. J. gen. Physiol. 11, 57–70 (1927).

198. McDowell, E.C., Gates, W.H., McDowell, C.G.: The influence of the quantity of nutrition upon the growth of the suckling mouse. J. gen. Physiol. 13, 529–545 (1930).

199. McLaren, A.: Genetics and environmental effects on foetal and placental growth in mice. J. Reprod. Fertil. 9, 79–98 (1965).

200. Ogana, T.: Comparative study on development in the stage of organogenesis in the mouse and rat. Congenit. Anomalies (Japan) 7, 27–31 (1967).

201. Reading, A.J.: Influence of room temperature on the growth of house mice. J. Mammal 47, 694–697 (1966).

202. Schumann, H.: Vergleichende Untersuchungen über das Wachstum von Ratten- und Mäuse-embryonen. Wilhelm Roux' Archiv 163, 325–333 (1969).

Addenda

Opera Generalia

Balls, M., Wild, A.E. (ed): The early development of mammals. London: Cambridge University Press 1975.

Oliver, G., Pineau, H.: Horizons de Streeter et áge embryonnaire. C.R. Ass. Anat. 47e Réun. Naples 1961, 113, 573–576 (1962).

Foster, H.L., Small, I.D., Fox, J.G. (ed): The mouse in biomedical research. New York: Academic Press 1983.

Preimplantation Period

Anderson, E., Hoppe, P.C., Whitten, W.K., Lee, G.S.: In vitro fertilization and early embryogenesis: A cytological analysis. J. Ultrastruct. Res. 50, 231–252 (1975).

Arguello, C., Martinez-Palomo, A.: Freeze-fracture morphology of gap junctions in the trophoblast of the mouse embryo. J. Ultrastruct. Res. 53, 271–283 (1975).

Bartel, H.: Electron microscopic observations of the inner cell mass of a mouse embryo. Acta anat. (Basel) 83, 89–301 (1972).

Batten, B.E., Albertini, D.F., Ducibella, T.: Patterns of organelle distribution in mouse embryos during preimplantation development. Am. J. Anat. 178, 65–71 (1987).

Bergström, S., Nilsson, O.: Embryo-endometrial relationship in the mouse during activation of the blastocyst by oestradiol. J. Reprod. Fert. 44, 117–120 (1975).

Brinster, R.L.: Parental glucose phosphate isomerase activity in three day mouse embryos. Biochem. Genet. 9, 187–191 (1973).

Calarco, P.G.: Cleavage (mouse) in S.E.M. Atlas of Mammalian Reproduction (Hafez, E.S.E., ed.), pp. 306–316. New York: Springer-Verlag 1975.

Calarco, P.G., Epstein, C.J.: Cell surface changes during preimplantation development in the mouse. Develop. Biol. 32, 208–213 (1973).

Ducibella, T., Albertini, D.F., Anderson, E., Biggers, J.D.: The preimplantation mammalian embryo: characterization of intercellular junctions and their appearance during development. Develop. Biol. 45, 231–250 (1975).

Ducibella, T., Anderson, E.: Cell shape and membrane changes in the eight-cell mouse embryo: prerequisites for morphogenesis of the blastocyst. Develop. Biol. 47, 45–58 (1975).

Fernandez, M.S., Izquierdo, L.: Blastocoel formation in half and double mouse embryos. Anat. Embryol. 160, 77–81 (1980).

Fleming, T.P., Goodall, H.: Endocytic traffic in trophectoderm and polarized blastomeres of the mouse preimplantation embryo. Anat. Rec. 216, 490–503 (1986).

Fleming, T.P., Pickering, S.J., Maro, B.: The generation of cell surface polarity in mouse 8-cell blastomeres: the role of cortical microfilaments analyzed using Cytochalasin D. J. Embryol. exp. Morph. 95, 169–191 (1986).

Fleming, T.P., Warren, P.D., Chisholm, J.C., Johnson, M.H.: Trophectodermal processes regulate the expression of totipotency within the inner cell mass of the mouse expanding blastocyst. J. Embryol. exp. Morph. 84, 63–90 (1984).

Gardner, R.L., Johnson, M.H.: Investigation of early mammalian development using interspecific chimaeras between rat and mouse. Nature New Biology 246, 86–89 (1973).

Goodall, H.: Manipulation of gap junctional communication during compaction of the mouse early embryo. J. Embryol. exp. Morph. 91, 283–296 (1986).

Hillman, N., Tasca, R.: Ultrastructural studies of the mouse blastocyst substages. Amer. J. Anat. 126, 151–174 (1969).

Houliston, E., Guilly, M.N., Courvalin, J.C., Maro, B.: Expression of nuclear lamins during mouse preimplantation development. Development 102, 251–258 (1988).

Johnson, M.H., Maro, B., Takeichi, M.: The role of cell adhesion in the synchronization and orientation of polarization in 8-cell mouse blastomeres. J. Embryol. exp. Morph. 93, 239–255 (1986).

Johnson, M.H., Pickering, S.J., Dhiman, A., Radcliffe, G.S., Maro, B.: Cytocortical organization during natural and prolonged mitosis of mouse 8-cell blastomeres. Development 102, 143–158 (1988).

Keneklis, T.P., Odartchenko, N.: Autoradiographic visualization of paternal chromosomes in mouse eggs. Nature 247, 215–216 (1974).

Kimber, S.J., McQueen, H.A., Bagley, P.R.: Fucosylated glycoconjugates in mouse preimplantation embryos. J. exp. Zool. 244, 395–408 (1987).

Lee, S.H., Ahuja, K.K., Gilburt, D.J., Whittingham, D.G.: The appearance of glycoconjugates associated with cortical granule release during mouse fertilization. Development 102, 595–604 (1988).

Levy, J.B., Johnson, M.H., Goodall, H., Maro, B.: The timing of compaction: Control of a major developmental transition in mouse early embryogenesis. J. Embryol. exp. Morph. 95, 213–237 (1986).

Maraldi, N.M., Monesi, V.: Ultrastructural changes from fertilization to blastulation in the mouse. Arch. Anat. micr. Morph. exp. 59, 361–382 (1970).

Maro, B., Johnson, M.H., Webb, M., Flach, G.: Mechanism of polar body formation in the mouse oocyte: an interaction between the chromosomes, the cytoskeleton and the plasma membrane. J. Embryol. exp. Morph. 92, 11–32 (1986).

McMahon, A., Fosten, M., Monk, M.: X-chromosome inactivation mosaicism in the three germ layers and the germ line of the mouse embryo. J. Embryol. exp. Morph. 74, 207–220 (1983).

Nadijcka, M., Hillman, N.: Ultrastructural studies of the mouse blastocyst substages. J. Embryol. exp. Morph. 32, 675–695 (1974).

Naeslund, G., Lundkvist, O., Nilsson, B.L.: Transmission electron microscopy of mouse blastocysts activated and growth-arrested in vivo and in vitro. Anat. Embryol. 159, 33–48 (1988).

Nilsson, B.O., Lundkvist, O.: Ultrastructural and histochemical changes of the mouse uterine epithelium on blastocyst activation for implantation. Anat. Embryol. 155, 311–321 (1979).

Pratt, H.P.M.: Membrane organization in the preimplantation mouse embryo. J. Embryol. exp. Morph. 90, 101–121 (1985).

Shirayoshi, Y., Okada, T.S., Takeichi, M.: The calcium-dependent cell-cell adhesion system regulates inner cell mass formation and cell surface polarization in early mouse development. Cell 35, 631–638 (1983).

Smith, L.J.: Embryonic axis orientation in the mouse and its correlation with blastocyst relationship to the uterus. II. Relationships from 4 1/4 to 9 1/2 days. J. Embryol. exp. Morph. 89, 15–35 (1985).

Smith, R.K.W., Johnson, M.H.: DNA replication and compaction in the cleaving embryo of the mouse. J. Embryol. exp. Morph. 89, 133–148 (1985).

Thompson, R.S., Zamboni, L.: Phagocytosis of supernumerary spermatozoa by two-cell mouse embryos. Anat. Rec. 178, 3–14 (1974).

Implantation and Fetal Membrane

Bell, K.E., Sherman, M.I.: Enzyme markers of mouse yolk differentiation. Develop. Biol. 33, 38–47 (1973).

Bellairs, R.: The primitive streak. Anat. Embryol. 174, 1–14 (1986).

Bergström, S., Nilsson, O.: Blastocyst attachment and early invasion during oestradiol-induced implantation in the mouse. Anat. Embryol. 149, 149–154 (1976).

Chavez, D.J.: Cell surface of mouse blastocysts at the trophectoderm-uterine interface during the adhesive stage of implantation. Am. J. Anat. 176, 153–158 (1986).

Doetschman, T.C., Eistetter, H., Katz, M., Schmidt, W., Kemler, R.: The in vitro development of blastocyst-derived embryonic stem cell lines: formation of visceral yolk sac, blood islands and myocardium. J. Embryol. exp. Morph. 87, 27–45 (1985).

El-Shershaby, A.M., Hinchcliff, J.R.: Epithelial autolysis during implantation of the mouse blastocyst: A light and electron microscopic study of dead cells and their fate. J. Embryol. exp. Morph. 31, 643–654 (1975).

Gardner, R.L., Papaioannou, V.E.: Origin of the ectoplacental cone and secondary giant cells in mouse blastocysts reconstituted from isolated trophoblast and inner cell mass. J. Embryol. exp. Morph. 30, 561–572 (1973).

Gearhart, J.D., Mintz, B.: Glucosephosphat isomerase subunit reassociation tests for maternal-fetal cell fusion in the mouse placenta. Develop. Biol. 29, 55–64 (1972).

Herken, R., Barrach, H.J.: Ultrastructural localization of type IV collagen and laminin in the seven-day old mouse embryo. Anat. Embryol. 171, 365–371 (1985).

Hernandez-Verdun, D.: Morphogenesis of the syncytium in the mouse placenta. Ultrastructural study. Cell Tiss. Res. 148, 381–396 (1974).

Hernandez-Verdun, D., Bouteille, M.: Nuclear differentiation during the course of syncytiogenesis in mouse trophoblast. J. Ultrastruct. Res. 57, 32–42 (1976).

Holland, P.W., Hogan, B.L.: Spatially restricted patterns of expression of the homeobox-containing gene Hox 2.1 during mouse embryogenesis. Development 102, 159–174 (1988).

Jolly, J., Ferester-Tadie, M.: Recherches sur l'oeuf du rat et de la souris. Arch. Anat. Micr. 32, 323–390 (1936).

Ishikawa, T., Seguchi, H.: Localization of Mg^{++}-dependent adenosine triphosphatase and alkaline phosphatase activities in the postimplantation mouse embryos in day 5 and 6. Anat. Embryol. 173, 7–11 (1985).

Krcek, J.P., Dickson, A.D., Biddle, F.G.: Numbers of metrial gland cells in the placental labyrinth of congenic resistant and inbred strains of mice, with observations on the size of the labyrinth. J. Anat. 140, 545–550 (1985).

Martello, E.M.V.G., Abrahamsom, P.A.: Collagen distribution in the mouse endometrium during decidualization. Acta anat. 127, 146–150 (1986).

Poelmann, R.E.: An ultrastructural study of implanting mouse blastocysts: coated vesicles and epithelium formation. J. Anat. 119, 421–434 (1975).

Rossant, J.: Investigation of the determinative state of the mouse inner cell mass. J. Embryol. exp. Morph. 33, 979–1001 (1975).

Searle, R.F., Jenkins, E.J.: Immunogenicity of mouse trophoblast and embryonic sac. Nature 255, 719–720 (1975).

Sherman, M.I., Kang, H.S.: DNA polymerase in mid-gestation mouse embryo, trophoblast, and decidua. Develop. Biol. 34, 200–210 (1973).

Solter, D., Damjanov, I., Skreb, N.: Ultrastructure of mouse egg cylinder. Z. Anat. Entwickl.-Gesch. 132, 291–298 (1970).

Smith, A.F., Wilson, I.B.: Cell interaction at the maternal-embryonic interface during implantation in the mouse. Cell and tissue Res. 152, 525–513 (1974).

Smith, M.S.R.: Changes in distribution of alkaline phosphatase during early implantation and development of the mouse. Austral. J. Biol. Sci. 26, 209–217 (1973).

Sobotta, J.: Die Entwicklung des Eies der Maus vom ersten Auftreten des Mesoderms an bis zur Ausbildung der Embronalanlage und dem Auftreten der Allantois. Arch. mikr. Anat. 78, 271–352 (1911).

Stewart, J., Peel, S.: The differentiation of the decidua and the distribution of metrial gland cells in the pregnant mouse uterus. Cell Tiss. Res. 187, 167–179 (1978).

Varmuza, S., Prideaux, V., Kothary, R., Rossant, J.: Polytene chromosomes in mouse trophoblast giant cells. Development 102, 127–134 (1988).

Blood and Cardiovascular System

Böck, P.: Das Glomus caroticum der Maus. Erg. Anat. u. Entwickl.-Gesch. 48, Part 1. Berlin: Springer 1973.

Borowski, R.: Elektronenmikroskopische Untersuchungen über den Wandaufbau der V. cardinalis post. bei Mäuseembryonen der Tage 10 und 11. Z. Anat. Entwickl.-Gesch. 140, 61–72 (1973).

Bugge, J.: The contribution of the stapedial artery to the cephalic arterial supply in muroid rodents. Acta anat. (Basel) 76, 313–336 (1970).

Cline, M.J., Moore, M.A.S.: Embryonic origin of the mouse macrophage. Blood 39, 942–849 (1972).

Furth, R. Van, Hirsch, J.G., Fedorko, M.E.: Morphology and peroxidase cytochemistry of mouse promonocytes, monocytes and macrophages. J. exp. Med. 132, 794–812 (1970).

Hollands, P.: Differentiation of haematopoetic stem cells from mouse blastocysts grown in vitro. Development 102, 135–142.

Hurle, J.M.: The development of the semilunar valves of the mouse. Anat. Embryol. 160, 83–92 (1980).

Jones, R.O.: Ultrastructural analysis of hepatic haematopoesis in the foetal mouse. J. Anat. (London) 107, 301–314 (1970).

Kazunobu, S., Kendall, M.D.: The morphology of the haematopoetic cells of the yolk sac in mice with particular reference to nucleolar changes. J. Anat. 140, 279–296 (1985).

Mierop, L.H.S. Van, Gessner, J.H.: The morphologic development of the sinoatrial node in the mouse. Am. J. Cardiol. 25, 204–212 (1970).

Navaratnam, V., Kaufmann, M.H., Skepper, J.N., Barton, S., Gutbridge, K.M.: Differentiation of the cardial rudiment of mouse embryos: an ultrastructural study including freeze-fracture replication. J. Anat. 146, 65–86 (1986).

Sasaki, K., Matsumura, G.: Haemopoetic cells of yolk sac and liver in the mouse embryo: a light and electron microscopic study. J. Anat. 148, 87–98 (1986).

Viragh, S., Challice, C.E.: Origin and differentiation of cardiac muscle cells in the mouse. J. Ultrastructure Res. 42, 1–24 (1973).

Viragh, S., Challice, C.E.: The development of the conductive system in the mouse embryo heart. Develop. Biol. 56, 397–411 (1977).

Viragh, S., Challice, C.E.: The origin of the epicardium and the embryonic myocardial circulation in the mouse. Anat. Rec. 201, 157–168 (1981).

Lymph Nodes, Thymus, Spleen

Abe, K., Ito, T.: Fine structure of small lymphocytes in the thymus of the mouse. Qualitative and quantitative analysis by electron microscope. Z. Zellforsch. 110, 321–335 (1970).

Bryant, B.J.: Renewal and fate in the mammalian thymus: mechanisms and interferences of thymokinetics. Europ. J. Immunol. 2, 38–45 (1972).

Groscurth, P., Kistler, G.: Histogenese des Immunsystems der "nude" Maus. IV. Ultrastruktur der Thymusanlage 12- und 13-tägiger Embryonen. Beitr. Path. 156, 359–375 (1975).

Kingston, R., Jenkinson, E.J., Owen, J.J.T.: Characterization of stroma cell populations in the developing thymus of normal and nude mice. Eur. J. Immunol. 14, 1052–1056 (1984).

Kowala, M.C., Schoefl, G.J.: The popliteal lymph node of the mouse: internal architecture, vascular distribution and lymphatic supply. J. Anat. 148, 25–46 (1986).

Papiernik, M., Nabarra, B.: Thymic reticulum in mice I. Cellular ultrastructure in vitro and functional role. Thymus 3, 345–358 (1981).

Zinkernagel, R.M.: Thymus and lymphopoetic cells: their role in T cell maturation, in selection of T cell restriction-specificity and in H-2-linked IR gene control. Immunol. Rev. 42, 224–270 (1978).

Miller, J.F.A.P., Mitchell, G.F.: Thymus and antigen-reactive cells. Transpl. Rev. 1, 3–42 (1969).

Owen, J.J.T., Raff, M.C.: Studies on the differentiation of thymus-derived lymphocytes. J. exp. Med. 132, 1216–1232 (1970).

Röpke, C., Jörgensen, O., Claesson, M.H.: Histochemical studies of high-endothelial venules of lymph nodes and Peyer's patches in the mouse. Z. Zellforsch. 131, 287–298 (1972).

Simpson, L.O.: Thymus weight changes during the early postnatal period in mice. Am. J. Anat. 138, 133–138 (1973).

Matter, A.: Morphological definition of thymocyte subpopulations. Cell Tiss. Res. 158, 319–332 (1975).

Van Deurs, B., Röpke, C.: The postnatal development of high-endothelial venules in the lymph nodes of mice. Anat. Rec. 181, 659–678 (1975).

Palate and Respiratory Tract

Breipohl, W.: Licht- und elektronenmikroskopische Befunde zur Struktur der Bowmanschen Drüsen im Riechepithel der weissen Maus. Z. Zellf. 131, 329–346 (1972).

Brinkley, L.L., Bookstein, F.L.: Cell distribution during mouse secondary palate closure II. Mesenchymal cells. J. Embryol. exp. Morph. 96, 111–130 (1986).

Hatasa, K., Nakamura. T.: Electron microscopic observations of lung alveolar epithelial cells of normal young mice with special reference to formation and secretion of osmiophilic lamellar bodies. Z. Zellforsch. 68, 266–277 (1965).

Knudsen, T.B., Bullert, R.F., Zimmerman, E.F.: Histochemical localization of glycosaminoglycans during morphogenesis of the secondary palate in mice. Anat. Embryol. 173, 137–142 (1985).

Stewart, J.: Granulated metrial cells in the lungs of mice in pregnancy and pseudo-pregnancy. J. Anat. 140, 551–564 (1985).

Ten Have-Opbroek, A.A.W.: The structural composition of the pulmonary acinus in the mouse. A scanning electron microscopic and developmental-biological analysis. Anat. Embryol. 174, 49–57 (1986).

Woodside, G.L., Dalton, A.J.: The ultrastructure of lung tissue from newborn and embryo mice. J. Ultrastruct. Res. 2, 28–54 (1958).

Yasuda, Y., Fujimoto, T.: The anterior half of mouse palatal shelf is elevated by a remodeling process. Acta Anat. 125, 37–41 (1986).

Oral Cavity

Berkman, M.D., Kronman, J.H.: A histochemical study of the effects of castration and testosterone administration on the major salivary glands of Swiss mice. Acta anat. (Basel) 76, 200–219 (1970).

Gresik, E.W., McRae, E.K.: The postnatal development of the sexually dimorphic duct system and of amylase activity in the submandibular glands of mice. Cell. Tiss. Res. 157, 411–428 (1975).

Gröneberg, H.: Exocrine glands and the Chievitz organ of some mouse mutants. J. Embryol. exp. Morph. 25, 247–261 (1971).

Nakano, T., Muto, H.: Anatomical observations in the pharynx of the mouse with special reference to the nasopharyngeal hiatus (Wood Jones). Acta anat. 121, 174–152 (1985).

McCulloch, C.A.G.: Progenitor cell populations in the periodontal ligament of mice. Anat. Rec. 211, 258–262 (1985).

Poelmann, R.E., Dubois, S.V., Hermsen, C., Smits-Van Prooije, A.E., Vermeij-Keers, C.H.R.: Cell degeneration and mitosis in the buccopharyngeal and branchial membranes in the mouse embryo. Anat. Embryol. 171, 187–192 (1985).

Wigglesworth, D.J., Longmore, G.A., Kuc, J.M., Murdoch, C.: Early dentinogenesis in mice: von Korff fibres and their possible significance. Acta Anat. 127, 151–160 (1986).

Intestinal Tract

Borghese, E., Laj, M., Dicaterino, B.: Acinar ultrastructure of the submandibular gland of the Mus musculus during embryonic development. Cell Tiss. Res. 150, 425–442 (1974).

Cheng, H., Bjerknes, M.: Whole population cell kinetics and postnatal development in the mouse intestinal epithelium. Anat. Rec. 211, 420–426 (1985).

Cockroft, D.L.: Regional and temporal differences in the parietal endoderm of the midgestation mouse embryo. J. Anat. 145, 35–48 (1986).

Coughlin, M.D.: Early development of parasympathetic nerves in the mouse submandibular gland. Develop. Biol. 43, 123–139 (1975).

Perissel, B., Malet, P., Pourhadi, R.: Différenciation des jonctions intrahépatocytaires chez la souris au cours de la période foetale. Bull. Assoc. des Anatomistes 58, 397–406 (1973).

Rothman, T.P., Tennyson, V.M., Gershon, M.D.: Colonization of the bowel by the precursors of enteric ganglia: Studies of normal and congenitally aganglionic mutant mice. J. comp. Neur. 252, 493–506 (1986).

Webster, W.: Embryogenesis of the enteric ganglia in normal mice and in mice that develop congenital aganglionic megacolon. J. Embryol. exp. Morph. 30, 573–585 (1973).

Urogenital Tract

Becker, K.: Paraganglienzellen im Ganglion cervicale uteri der Maus. Z. Zellforsch. 130, 249–261 (1972).

Bourgoyne, P.S., Buehr, M., Koopman, P., Rossant, J., McLaren, A.: Cell-autonomous action of the testis-determining gene: Sertoli cells are exclusively XY in XX–XY chimaeric mouse testis. Development 101, 127–134 (1988).

Bryan, J.H.D., Wolosewick, J.J.: Spermatogenesis revisited. II. Ultrastructural studies of spermiogenesis in multinucleate spermatides of the mouse. Z. Zellforsch. 138, 295–298 (1973).

Burkett, B.N., Schulte, B.A., Spicer, S.S.: Histochemical evaluation of glycoconjugates in the male reproductive tract with lectin-horseradish peroxidase conjugates. Am. J. Anat. 178, 11–29 (1987).

Cunha, G.R.: Peristaltic contraction of the murine urogenital sinus. Anat. Rec. 177, 561–568 (1973).

Cunha, G.R.: Stromal induction and specification of morphogenesis and cytodifferentiation of the Müllerian ducts and urogenital sinus during development of the uterus and vagina in mice. J. exp. Zool. 196, 361–370 (1976).

Czaker, R.: Relative position of constitutive heterochromatin and of nucleolar structures during mouse spermiogenesis. Anat. Embryol. 175, 467–475 (1987).

Deburlet, H.M., De Ruiter, H.J.: Zur Entwicklung und Morphologie des Säugerhodens I. Der Hoden von mus musculus. Anatomische Hefte 59, 325–382 (1921).

Dooher, G.B., Bennett, D.: Fine structural observations on the development of the sperm head in the mouse. Am. J. Anat. 136, 339–362 (1973).

Forsberg, J.G., Abro, A.: Ultrastructural studies on cell degeneration in the mouse uterovaginal anlage. Acta anat. 85, 353–367 (1973).

Goodfellow, P.N., Darling, S.M.: Genetics of sex determination in man and mouse. Development 102, 251–258 (1988).

Jeon, K.W., Kennedy, J.R.: The primordial germ cells in early mouse embryos: light and electron microscopic studies. Develop. Biol. 31, 275–284 (1973).

Jost, S.P.: Postnatal growth of the mouse bladder. J. Anat. 143, 39–44 (1985).

Kluin, P.M., Kramer, M.F., De Rooij, D.G.: Proliferation of spermatogonia and Sertoli cells in maturing mice. Anat. Embryol. 169, 73–78 (1984).

Kriz, W., Koepsell, H.: The structural organization of the mouse kidney. Z. Anat. Entwickl.-Gesch. 144, 137–164 (1974).

Mauch, R.B., Tiedemann, K.U., Drews, U.: The vagina is formed by downgrowth of Wolffian and Müllerian ducts. Graphical reconstructions from normal and Tfm mouse embryos. Anat. Embryol. 172, 75–87 (1985).

Mitchell, P.A., Burghardt, R.C.: The ontogeny of nexuses (gap junctions) in the ovary of the fetal mouse. Anat. Rec. 214, 283–288 (1986).

Murakami, R.: A histological study of development of the penis of wild-type and androgen-insensitive mice. J. Anat. 153, 223–232 (1987).

Odor, D.L., Blandau, R.J.: Ultrastructural studies on fetal and early postnatal mouse ovaries. II. Cytodifferentiation. Am. J. Anat. 125, 177–216 (1969).

Redi, C.A., Garagna, S., Hilscher, B., Winking, H.: The effects of some Robertsonian chromosome combinations on the seminiferous epithelium of the mouse. J. Embryol. exp. Morph. 85, 1–19 (1985).

Spiegelman, M., Bennet, D.: A light- and electron microscopic study of primordial germ cells in the early mouse embryo. J. Embryol. exp. Morph. 30, 97–118 (1973).

Endocrine Glands

Broecker, E.B.: Die Lipoidtropfen in der Nebennierenrinde der weiblichen Maus und Beziehungen ihrer Grössenverteilung zum Zyklus. Z. Zellforsch. 113, 188–202 (1971).

Cordier, A.C., Haumoont, S.M.: Development of thymus, parathyroids, and ultimo-branchial bodies in NMRI and nude mice. Am. J. Anat. 157, 227–263 (1980).

Emerman, J.T., Vogl, W.: Cell size and shape changes in the myoepithelium of the mammary gland during differentiation. Anat. Rec. 216, 405–415 (1986).

Eurenius, L., Jarskär, R.: Electron microscope studies on the development of the external zone of the mouse median eminence. Z. Zellforsch. 122, 488–502 (1971).

Eurenius, L., Jarskär, R.: Electron microscopy of neurosecretory nerve fibres in the neural lobe of the embryonic mouse. Cell Tiss. Res. 149, 333–347 (1974).

Fernholm, M.: On the development of the sympathetic chain and the adrenal medulla in the mouse. Z. Anat. Entwickl.-Gesch. 133, 305–317 (1971).

Garweg, G., Kinsey, J., Brinkmann, H.: Markierung der juxta medullären X-Zone in der Nebenniere der Maus mit L-Cystein-S^{35}. Z. Anat. Entwickl.-Gesch. 134, 186–199 (1971).

Gomez-Dumm, C.L.A., Echave-Llanos, J.M.: Further studies on the ultrastructure of the pars distalis of the male mouse hypophysis. Acta anat. 82, 254–266 (1972).

Hirokawa, N., Ishikawa, H.: Electron microscopic observations on postnatal development of the X-zone on mouse adrenal cortex. Z. Anat. Entwickl.-Gesch. 144, 1–18 (1974).

Monkhouse, W.S., Chell, J.: The effect of hydrocortisone on the para-aortic body of the newborn mouse: an in vivo fraction of labelled mitoses study. J. Anat. 150, 211–218 (1987).

Müntener, M., Theiler, K.: Die Entwicklung der Nebennieren der Maus. II. Postnatale Entwicklung. Z. Anat. Entwickl.-Gesch. 144, 205–214 (1974).

Peel, S. Stewart, J.: Oestrogen and the differentiation of granulated metrial gland cells in chimeric mice. J. Anat. 144, 181–188 (1986).

Stoeckel, M.E., Dellmann, H.D., Porte, A., Gertner, C.: The rostral zone of the intermediate lobe of the mouse hypophysis, a zone of particular concentration of corticotrophic cells. Z. Zellforsch. 122, 310–322 (1971).

Theiler, K., Müntener, M.: Die Entwicklung der Nebennieren der Maus. I. Pränatale Entwicklung. Z. Anat. Entwickl.-Gesch. 144, 195–204 (1974).

Treilhou-Lahiville, F., Beaumont, A.: Etude ultrastructurale du corps ultimo-branchial et de l' épithélium pharyngien du foetus de souris á partir du 11éme jour de vie intra-uterine. J. Ultrastruct. Res. 50, 387–403 (1975).

Wilson, D.B.: Distribution of H^3-Thymidin in the postnatal hypophysis of the C57BL mouse. Acta anat. 126, 121–126 (1986).

Wollman, S.H., Hilfer, S.R.: Embryologic origin of the various epithelial cell types in the second kind of thyroid follicle in the C3H mouse. Anat. Rec. 191, 111–122 (1978).

Brain, Sensory Organs, Skin

Beauvillain, J.C.: Structure fine de l' éminence médiane de souris au cours de son ontogénèse. Z. Zellforsch. 139, 201–215 (1973).

Bhattacharjee, J., Sanyal, S.: Developmental origin and early differentiation of retinal Müller cells in mice. J. Anat. 120, 367–372 (1975).

Caviness, V.S.: Time of neuron origin in the hippocampus and dentate gyrus of normal and reeler mutant mice: an autoradiographic analysis. J. comp. Neurol. 151, 113–120 (1973).

Chan, W.Y., Tam, P.P.L.: The histogenetic potential of neural plate cells of early-somite stage mouse embryos. J. Embryol. exp. Morph. 96, 183–193 (1986).

Chan, W.Y., Tam, P.P.L.: A morphological and experimental study of the mesencephalic neural crest cells in the mouse embryo using wheat germ agglutinin-gold conjugate as the cell marker. Development 102, 427–442 (1988).

Cooper, N.G.F., Steindler, D.A.: Lectins demarcate the barrel subfield in the somato-sensory cortex of the early postnatal mouse. J. comp. Neurol. 249, 157–169 (1986).

Cuschieri, A., Bannister, L.H.: The development of the olfactory mucosa in the mouse: electron microscopy. J. Anat. 119, 471–498 (1975).

Davies, A.M., Lumsden, A.G.S.: Fasciculation in the early mouse trigeminal nerve is not ordered in relation to the emerging pattern of whisker follicles. J. comp. Neurol. 253, 13–24 (1986).

Derer, P., Caviness, V.S., Sidman, R.L.: Early cortical histogenesis in the primary olfactory cortex of the mouse. Brain Res. 123, 27–40 (1977).

Dry, F.W.: The coat of the mouse. J. Genet. 16, 287–340 (1926).

Dubrul, E.F.: Fine structure of epidermal differentiation in the mouse . J. exp. Zool. 181, 145–158 (1972).

Edwards, M.A., Caviness, V.S., Schneider, G.E.: Development of cell and fiber lamination in the mouse superior colliculus. J. comp. Neurol. 248, 395–409 (1986).

Ehrenbrand, F.: Über ein Paraganglion vestibulare bei der Maus. Z. Anat. Entwickl.-Gesch. 137, 285–300 (1972).

Fentress, J.C., Standfield, B.B., Cowan, W.M.: Observations on the development of the striatum in mice and rats. Anat. Embryol. 163, 275–298 (1981).

Fisher, L.J.: Development of synaptic arrays in the inner plexiform layer of neonatal mouse retina. J. comp. Neurol. 187, 359–372 (1979).

Fujimiya, M., Kimura, H., Maeda, T.: Postnatal development of serotonin nerve fibres in the somatosensory cortex of mice studied by immunohistochemistry. J. comp. Neurol. 246, 191–201 (1986).

Geelan, J.A.G., Langman, J.: Closure of the neural tube in the cephalic region of the mouse embryo. Anat. Rec. 189, 625–640 (1977).

Goffinet, A.M., Lyon, G.: Early histogenesis in the mouse cerebral cortex: a Golgy study. Neurosci. Lett. 14, 61–66 (1979).

Haustein, J.: On the ultrastructure of the developing and adult mouse corneal stroma. Anat. Embryol. 168, 291–305 (1983).

Hearing, V.J., Phillips, P., Lutzner, M.A.: The fine structure of melanogenesis in coat color mutants of the mouse. J. Ultrastruct. Res. 43, 88–106 (1973).

Hinds, J.W., Hinds, P.L.: Early ganglion cell differentiation in the mouse retina: An electron microscopic analysis utilizing serial sections. Develop. Biol. 37, 381–416 (1974).

Hinds, J.W., Hinds, P.L.: Early development of amacrine cells in the mouse retina. An electron microscopic, serial section analysis. J. comp. Neurol. 179, 277–300 (1978).

Hinds, J.W., Ruffett, T.: Cell proliferation in the neural tube: An electron microscopic and Golgi analysis in the mouse cerebral vesicle. Z. Zellforsch. 115, 226–264 (1971).

Jacobsen, A.G., Tam, P.P.L.: Cephalic neurulation in the mouse embryo analyzed by SEM and morphometry. Anat. Rec. 203, 375–396 (1982).

Innes, P.B.: The ultrastructure of the early cephalic neural crest cell migration in the mouse. Anat. Embryol. 172, 33–38 (1985).

Lavail, M.M.: Kinetics of rod outer segment renewal in the developing mouse retina. J. Cell Biol. 58, 650–661 (1973).

Lehmann, A.: Atlas stereotaxique du cerveau de la souris. Paris: Editions du Centre Nationale de la Recherche Scientifique, 15 quai Anatole France, 75700 Paris 1975.

Li, C.W., Van de Water, T.R.: The fate mapping of the eleventh and twelfths day mouse otocyst: An in vitro study of the sites of origin of the embryonic inner ear sensory structures. J. Morph. 157, 249–267 (1978).

Lund, R.D., Perry, V.H., Lagenaur, C.F.: Cell surface changes in the developing optic nerve of mice. J. comp. Neurol. 247, 439–446 (1986).

Lyon, M.F.: The development of the otoliths of the mouse. J. Embryol. exp. Morph. 3, 213–229 (1955).

Martins-Green, M., Erickson, C.A.: Development of neural tube basal lamina during neurulation and neural crest cell emigration in the trunk of the mouse embryo. J. Embryol. exp. Morph. 98, 219–236 (1986).

Mayer, T.C.: The migratory pathway of neural crest cells into the skin of mouse embryos. Develop. Biol. 34, 39–46 (1973).

Mbiene, J.P., Sans, A.: Differentiation and maturation of the sensory hair bundles in the fetal and postnatal vestibular receptors of the mouse: A scanning electron microscopy study. J. comp. Neurol. 254, 271–278 (1986).

Miale, I.L., Sidman, R.L.: An autoradiographic analysis of histogenesis in the mouse cerebellum. Exp. Neurol. 4, 227–296 (1961).

Nichols, D.H.: Formation and distribution of neural crest mesenchyme to the first pharyngeal arch region of the mouse embryo. Am. J. Anat. 176, 221–232 (1986).

Pei, Y.F., Rhodin, J.A.G.: The prenatal development of the mouse eye. Anat. Rec. 168, 105–126 (1970).

Reams, W.M., Jr., Tomkins, S.P.: A developmental study of murine epidermal Langhans cells. Develop. Biol. 31, 114–123 (1973).

Sakai, Y.: Neurulation in the mouse. I. The ontogenesis of neural segments and the determination of topographical regions in a central nervous system. Anat. Rec. 218, 450–457 (1987).

Schoenwolf, F.G.: Histological and ultrastructural studies of secondary neurulation in mouse embryos. Am. J. Anat. 169, 361–376 (1984).

Schlüter, G.: Ultrastructural observations on cell necrosis during formation of the neural tube in mouse embryos. Z. Anat. Entwickl.-Gesch. 141, 251–264 (1973).

Sheer, A.E.: The embryonic and postnatal development of the inner ear of the mouse. Acta Otolaryngol. (Stockholm) Suppl. 285, 1–77 (1971).

Shoukimas, G., Hinds, J.W.: The development of the cerebral cortex in the embryonic mouse: An electron microscopic serial section analysis. J. comp. Neurol. 179, 795–830 (1978).

Sidman, R.L., Angevine, J.B., Pierce, E.T.: Atlas of the mouse brain and spinal cord. Berlin-Heidelberg-New York: Springer-Verlag 1971.

Silvers, W.K.: The coat colors of the mice. Berlin-Heidelberg-New York: Springer-Verlag 1979.

Smart, I.H.M.: A localized growth zone in the wall of the developing mouse telencaphalon. J. Anat. 140, 397–402 (1985).

Stanfield, B.B., Cowan, W.M.: The development of the hippocampus and dentate gyrus in normal and reeler mice. J. comp. Neurol. 185, 423–460 (1979).

Sternberg, J., Kimber, S.J.: The relationship between emerging neural crest cells and basement membranes in the trunk of the mouse embryo: TEM and immunocytochemical study. J. Embryol. exp. Morph. 98, 261–268 (1986).

Sturrock, R.R.: Age-related changes in the number of myelinated axons and glial cells in the anterior and posterior limbs of the mouse anterior commissure. J. Anat. 150, 111–128 (1987).

Sturrock, R.R.: An ultrastructural study of the development of leptomeningeal macrophages in the mouse and rabbit. J. Anat. 156, 207–216 (1988).

Taber, P.E.: Histogenesis of the dorsal and ventral cochlear nuclei in the mouse. An autoradiographic study. J. comp. Neurol. 131, 27–54 (1967).

Tam, P.P.L., Kwong, W.H.: A study on the pattern of alkaline phosphatase activity correlated with observations on silver-impregnated structures in the developing mouse brain. J. Anat. 150, 169–180 (1987).

Theiler, K., Sweet, H.O.: Low set ears (Lse), a new mutation of the house mouse. Anat. Embryol. 175, 241–246 (1986).

Werwoerd, C.D.A., Van Oostrom, C.G.: Cephalic neural crest and placodes. Advances in Anat., Embryol. and Cell Biol. Berlin-Heidelberg-New York: Springer-Verlag 1979.

Webster, E.H., Searl, R.L., Hilfer, S.R., Zwaan, J.: Accumulation and distribution of sulfated materials in the maturing mouse lens capsule. Anat. Rec. 218, 329–337 (1987).

Wilson, D.B., Hendrickx, A.G.: A comparative analysis of (H^3) Thymidine labelling in the embryonic tectum of the Rhesus Monkey (Macaca mulatta) and C57BL mouse. Anat. Embryol. 164, 277–285 (1982).

Woodhams, E., Basco, E., Hajos, F., Csillag, A., Balazs, R.: Radial glia in the developing mouse cerebral cortex and hippocampus. Anat. Embryol. 163, 331–343 (1981).

Wrenn, J.T., Wessells, N.K.: An ultrastructural study of lens invagination in the mouse. J. exp. Zool. 171, 359–368 (1969).

Young, R.W.: Cell differentiation in the retina of the mouse. Anat. Rec. 212, 199–205 (1985).

Zilles, K., Wingert, F.: Biometrische Analyse der Frischvolumina des Nucleus ruber einer ontogenetische Reihe von Albinomäusen. Z. Anat. Entwickl.-Gesch. 138, 215–226 (1972).

Skeletal System, Musculature

Cole, A.A., Wezeman, H.: Cytochemical localization of Tartrate-resistant acid phosphatase, alkaline phosphatase, and nonspecific esterase in perivascular cells of cartilage canals in the developing mouse epiphysis. Am. J. Anat. 180, 237–242 (1987).

Dawes, B.: The development of the vertebral column in mammals as illustrated by its development in Mus musculus. Philos. Trans. R. Soc. Lond. (Biol.) 218, 115–170 (1930).

Furtwängler, J.A., Hall, S.H., Koskinen-Moffett, L.K.: Structural morphogenesis in the mouse calvaria: the role of apophysis. Acta anat. 124, 74–80 (1985).

Gearhart, J.D., Mintz, B.: Clonal origins of somites and their muscle derivatives: evidence from allophenic mice. Develop. Biol. 29, 27–37 (1972).

Jurand, A.: Some aspects of the development of the notochord in mouse embryos. J. Embryol. exp. Morph. 32, 1–33 (1974).

Maeda, N., Osawa, K., Masuda, T., Hakeda, Y., Kumegana, M.: Postnatal development of the anulospiral endings of Ia-fibres in muscle spindles of mice. Acta anat. 124, 42–46 (1985).

Platzer, A.C.: The ultrastructure of normal myogenesis in the limb of the mouse. Anat. Rec. 190, 639–658 (1978).

Sensenig, E.C.: The origin of the vertebral column in the deermouse, Peromyxcus maniculatus rufinus. Anat. Rec. 86, 123–141 (1943).

Tam, P.P.: A study on the pattern of prospective somites in the presomitic mesoderm of mouse embryos. J. Embryol. exp. Morph. 92, 269–285 (1986).

Tam, P.P.L., Meier, S.: The establishment of a somitomeric pattern in the mesoderm of the gastrulating mouse embryo. Am. J. Anat. 164, 209–225 (1982).

Theiler, K.: Vertebral malformations. Experiments, genetics, development. Advances in Anat. Embryol. and Cell Biol., 112, Berlin-Heidelberg-New York: Springer-Verlag 1988.

Verbout, A.J.: The development of the vertebral column. Advances in Anat. Embryol. and Cell Biol. 90, Berlin-Heidelberg-New York: Springer-Verlag 1985.

Growth

Goedbloed, J.F.: The embryonic and postnatal growth of rat and mouse. I. The embryonic and early postnatal growth of the whole embryo. A model with exponential growth and sudden changes in growth rate. Acta anat. 82, 305–336 (1972).

Heinecke, H.: Embryologischer Parameter verschiedener Mäusestämme. Z. Versuchstierkunde 14, 154–171 (1972).

Hetherington, C.M.: The effect of parity on decidual, placental and fetal weight in the mouse. J. Reproduct. fertil. 28, 125–129 (1972).

Yamamura, H.: Individuelle Unterschiede des Entwicklungsstandes bei Embryonen der Maus (C57BL) in der frühen Phase der Organogenese. Wilhelm Roux' Archiv 162, 218–242 (1969).

Index

176

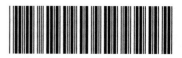